Single Port Gynecologic Laparoscopic and Robotic-Assisted Surgery

Edited by Greg Marchand

Published in London, United Kingdom

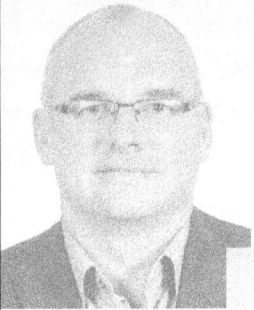
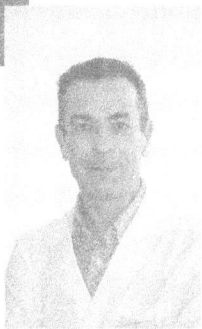
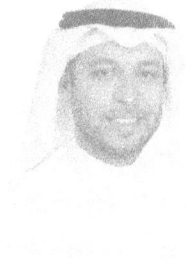
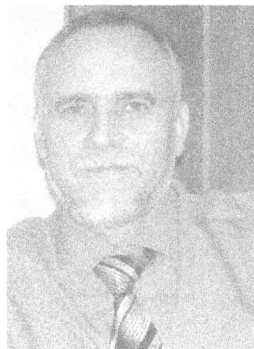
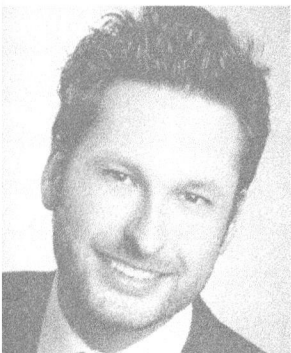
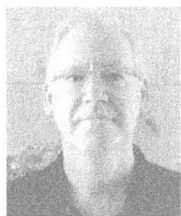
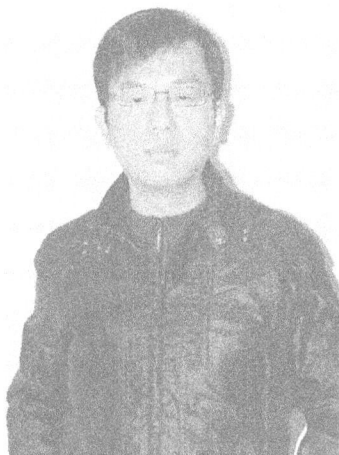

IntechOpen

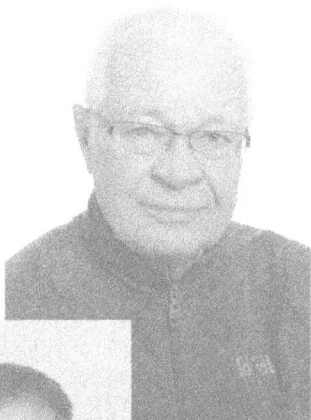
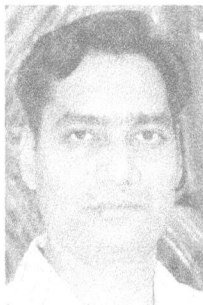
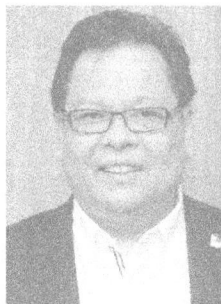
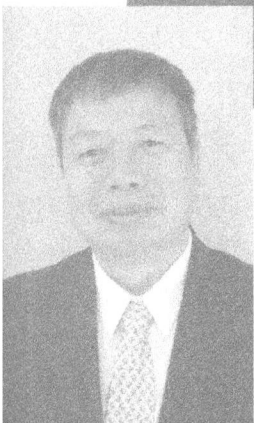
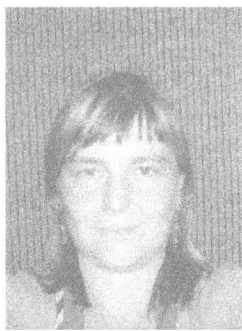
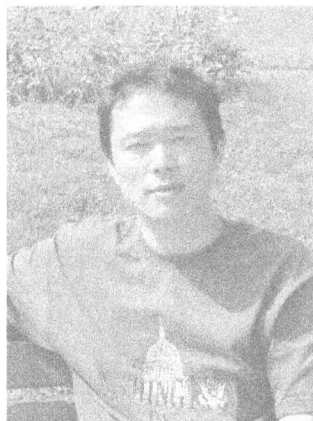

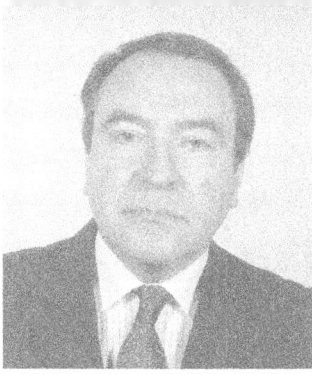

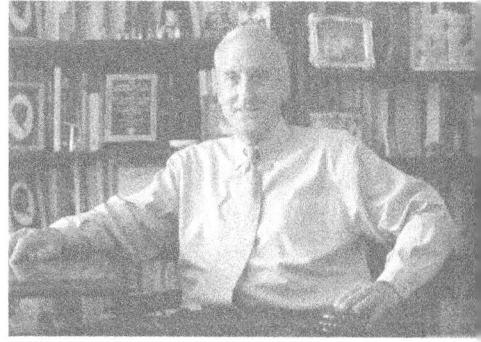

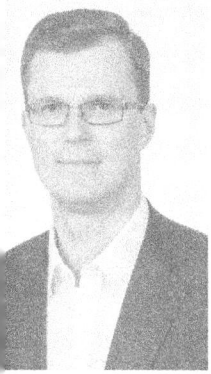

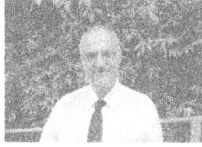

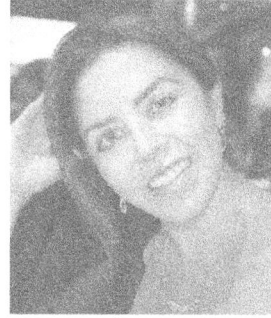

Supporting open minds since 2005

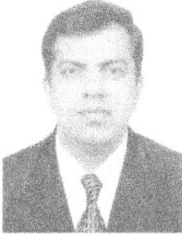

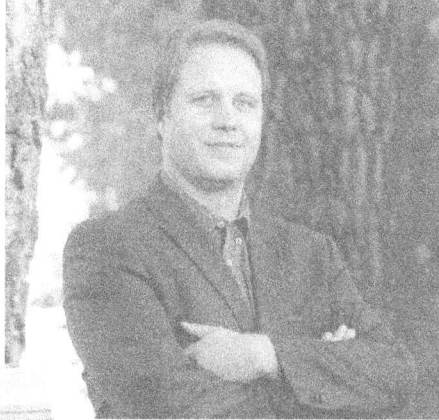

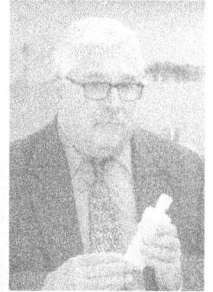

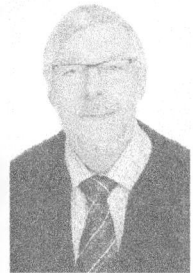

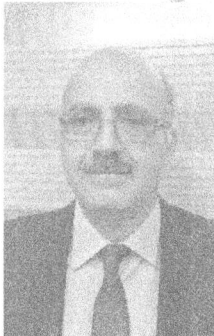

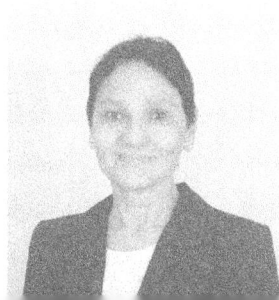

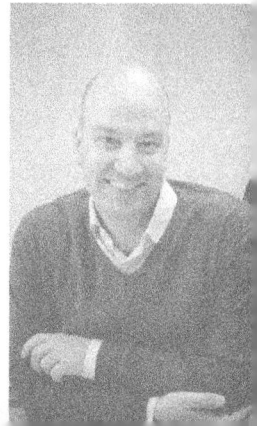

Single Port Gynecologic Laparoscopic and Robotic-Assisted Surgery
http://dx.doi.org/10.5772/intechopen.93283
Edited by Greg Marchand

Contributors
M. Luann Racher, Ann Marie Mercier, Alexander F. Burnett, Martha O. Rojo, Stephen Bush II, Conor J. Corcoran, Stephen H. Bush, Rene I. Luna, Michael L. Nimaroff, Eric Crihfield, John R. Wagner

Notice
Statements and opinions expressed in the chapters are these of the individual contributors and not necessarily those of the editors or publisher. No responsibility is accepted for the accuracy of information contained in the published chapters. The publisher assumes no responsibility for any damage or injury to persons or property arising out of the use of any materials, instructions, methods or ideas contained in the book.

First published in London, United Kingdom, 2021 by IntechOpen
IntechOpen is the global imprint of INTECHOPEN LIMITED, registered in England and Wales, registration number: 11086078, 5 Princes Gate Court, London, SW7 2QJ, United Kingdom
Printed in Croatia

British Library Cataloguing-in-Publication Data
A catalogue record for this book is available from the British Library

Additional hard and PDF copies can be obtained from orders@intechopen.com

Single Port Gynecologic Laparoscopic and Robotic-Assisted Surgery
Edited by Greg Marchand
p. cm.
Print ISBN 978-1-83880-251-6
Online ISBN 978-1-83881-033-7
eBook (PDF) ISBN 978-1-83881-034-4

We are IntechOpen,
the world's leading publisher of
Open Access books
Built by scientists, for scientists

5,400+
Open access books available

134,000+
International authors and editors

165M+
Downloads

Our authors are among the

156
Countries delivered to

Top 1%
most cited scientists

12.2%
Contributors from top 500 universities

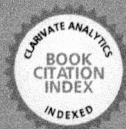

CLARIVATE ANALYTICS
BOOK
CITATION
INDEX
INDEXED

WEB OF SCIENCE™

Selection of our books indexed in the Book Citation Index
in Web of Science™ Core Collection (BKCI)

Interested in publishing with us?
Contact book.department@intechopen.com

Numbers displayed above are based on latest data collected.
For more information visit www.intechopen.com

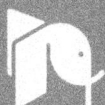

Meet the editor

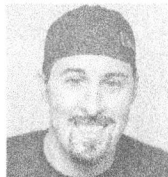

Dr. Greg Marchand is a board-certified OBGYN trained in minimally invasive gynecologic surgery. He is one of the few OBGYNs in the United States to be accredited as a Master Surgeon in Minimally Invasive Gynecologic Surgery. He is also a nationally sought-after expert for opinions in gynecology who has appeared on Today and Inside Edition, among other television shows. Dr. Marchand is the holder of several world records in gynecologic surgery, including a Guinness World Record in Laparoscopic Hysterectomy. As an inventor, Dr. Marchand holds several patents for surgical procedures and his techniques are taught at institutes of higher learning across the country. When not in the operating room, Dr. Marchand enjoys low-carb living and chasing his eight-year-old son Sebastian around.

Contents

Preface

Now is an exciting time in minimally invasive gynecologic surgery. In May 2021, we have had the first group of OBGYN's to receive a focused practice designation for Minimally Invasive Gynecologic Surgery. Currently, there are more than sixty fellowship programs in the United States for MIGS, split between the Society of Laparoendoscopic Surgeons (SLS) and the American Association of Gynecologic Laparoscopists (AAGL). Many would say we are on our way to becoming a separately boarded specialty. Our mission of providing the most minimally invasive care possible is well underway.

Also, an unexpected ally has shown its face in this battle. Enhanced Recovery After Surgery (ERAS) continues to be an important element in our artform. For a practice that is barely 20 years old, the amount of literature is extremely vast and very useful. All aspects of the preoperative and postoperative periods have been dissected, and minimally invasive surgeons can benefit from this data in almost all procedures. Surgeons and anesthesiologists can manipulate local anesthesia, patient diet, ambulation, and thrombotic prophylaxis. Even gum chewing has been included in regimens to speed patient recovery and decrease the pain and suffering of the surgical process. Many ERAS protocols are so individualized as to apply to one specific surgery. This may be the friend we've always wanted!

That is not to say that there are not challenges, the most serious of which has been the crisis of morcellation. Laparoscopic morcellation, when performed by skilled surgeons in appropriate circumstances, can be life-changing. I have seen it change a disabled invalid with a seven-pound uterus and serious comorbidities into a functional happy woman who walked out of a hospital she needed a wheelchair to get into just six hours earlier. Obviously, morcellation has been misused in situations where malignancy was likely, and even over-used in scenarios where uteri have been morcellated even after creating a colpotomy large enough to simply pull it out. As a result, patients have been harmed. Clearly, combining morcellation with an occult malignancy is a terrible event, but I will wager that "conversion to laparotomy," because of the lack of the ability to perform morcellation, has cost many more lives than upstaged leiomyosarcoma ever has. No one knows how many patients have died or remained debilitated the rest of their lives because of the surgeon's decision to create a midline vertical rather than morcellate. I believe there is close to 100 percent consensus among gynecologic surgeons today that laparoscopic morcellation should be reserved for special cases where vaginal removal is simply not feasible and laparotomy would pose a serious threat to the patient's life or speedy recovery. In those cases, with all reasonable measures taken, the procedure is a very valuable tool. Much like chemotherapy, however, if used on the wrong patient it can be harmful or deadly. In my opinion, we need the patient population to understand the foolishness of banning morcellation and bring careful judicious use of laparoscopic morcellation when indicated back into the mainstream of MIGS.

The inspiration for this book is the constant drive to provide patients with the most minimally invasive surgery possible. I was very blessed early on by several colleagues who share this drive. As a result, our discussions turned into an idea for a book, and before long we were finishing up this first edition.

Writing the book was a difficult task, as some of us wanted more of a direct surgical and anatomical guide, whereas others preferred a text that would give more of an overview of the subject without actual operating room value. The former was initially thought to be more valuable, however, the argument that nothing could replace a well-thought-out surgical good demonstrating video was also a concern. As for the latter, we hypothesized it would probably be a more popular text, but of less use on a day-to-day basis. In the end, we looked at what each chapter presented us and tried to pick the option that would best serve the reader. Some chapters resemble UpToDate articles, while others present more like instructional manuals. I hope we have reached the right balance.

We hope this text gives you some insight into the field of single-port gynecologic surgery and helps to form a consensus among surgeons and scholars of what techniques are the most effective, as well as what techniques are holding back the art and science of single-port surgery.

Every effort has been made to assure the reliability and value of the material in this book, and we are grateful that you are reading this first edition.

We are proud that you are on this journey with us and we are proud of where we are going. After all, aren't we just one port away from being right back at the TVH we started with?

I wish to thank Dr. Katelyn Sainz for helping me and putting up with me throughout the task of completing this book! I also extend a big thank you to all my researchers: Alexa King, Giovanna Brazil, Holly Ulibarri, Kelly Ware, Stacy Ruther, Julia Parise, Amanda Arroyo, and Sienna Anderson! I am also grateful to Dr. Ali Azadi, Dr. Hadia Awad, and Dr. Ahmed Taher. Finally, I have to mention Sebastian Snow Marchand, the smartest person I know. Thank you for teaching me so much.

Greg J. Marchand MD, FACS, FACOG, FICS
Fellowship Trained in Minimally Invasive Gynecologic Surgery,
Mesa, Arizona

Accredited Master Surgeon,
Minimally Invasive Gynecology,
Mesa, Arizona

Director,
Marchand Institute for Minimally Invasive Surgery,
Mesa, Arizona

Full Professor,
Washington University of Health and Science,
San Pedro, Belize

Associate Clinical Professor,
AT Still University,
College of Osteopathic Medicine,
Mesa, Arizona

Associate Clinical Professor,
Midwestern University,
College of Osteopathic Medicine,
Glendale, Arizona

Associate Clinical Professor,
IUHS,
Basseterre, Saint Kitts

Fundamentals of the Currently Available Single Port Abdominal Laparoscopic Gynecologic Systems and Utility in Minor Gynecologic Surgery

M. Luann Racher and Ann Marie Mercier

Abstract

Single incision laparoscopic surgery encompasses a plethora of techniques and styles. Single incision laparoscopy has demonstrated outcomes comparable to traditional multiport laparoscopy with the added benefit of improved cosmesis. This book chapter will review single incision surgery for minor gynecologic surgery, including adnexal surgical procedures and myomectomy. The chapter reviews available data in regard to outcomes in single incision laparoscopy. It also discusses the commercially available single incision surgical access systems, laparoscopes, and accessory instruments. Surgical techniques beneficial in single incision laparosocpy, including uterine manipulation, are also reviewed.

Keywords: single port, laparoscopy, SILS, LESS, single incision, minimally invasive, gynecology

1. Introduction

Single incision laparoscopic surgery encompasses a plethora of techniques and styles. Multiple names have been used to describe similar surgical techniques, including single incision laparoscopy (SILS), single port access surgery (SPA), laparoscopic endoscopic single site surgery (LESS), single laparoscopic incision transabdominal (SLIT), one-port umbilical surgery (OPUS), and natural orifice translumenal endoscopic surgery (NOTES). The purpose of this chapter is to review single incision surgery in minor gynecologic surgery and discuss currently available single incision surgical access systems, accessory instruments and surgical techniques in single incision gynecologic surgery.

2. Use of single port abdominal laparoscopy in minor gynecologic surgery

Female sterilization by tubal ligation was the first procedure performed by way of single incision laparoscopy in the late 1960s. Though gynecologists were the first surgeons to perform SILS, the technique was more readily adopted by urologists in the 1990s [1]. Now, more than 40 years since its development, single incision laparoscopy has become widespread in gynecologic surgery. Minor gynecologic procedures that have been performed by single incision include, but are not limited to: diagnostic laparoscopy, tubal sterilization (by both occlusion and partial or complete salpingectomy), management of ectopic pregnancy, ovarian cystectomy, oophorectomy, ovarian detorsion, oophoropexy and myomectomy. Adnexal surgeries, especially oophorectomy and ovarian cystectomy, are the most commonly performed minor gynecologic SILS procedures [2–4].

Single incision laparoscopy has a greater degree of difficulty than multiport laparoscopy, mainly due to reduction of triangulation (**Figure 1a, b**). In multi-port laparoscopy, ports may be placed in a triangular formation in Ref. to the target organ. Generally, the central optical trocar is placed 10-15 cm away from the target organ and accessory ports are placed laterally along an arc maintaining a similar distance from the target organ. Instruments are then commonly introduced at a 60 degree angle. A wide angle of manipulation, ideally between 45 and 75 degrees, results in the most efficient movements from the surgeon. Triangulation also allows for the appropriate traction and countertraction necessary to retract, dissect, ligate, and suture during a multiport laparoscopic procedure [5, 6].

With a narrow angle of triangulation, as in single incision laparoscopy, ergonomics become more limited. Surgical techniques, advanced uterine manipulation, articulating or prebent instruments, and angled or flexible laparoscopes can improve surgical constraints, but the degree of technical difficulty remains higher in single incision laparoscopy. Cross-triangulation, or the crossing of surgical instruments, may improve triangulation constraints [5, 6].

Most authors agree that between 5 and 30 cases are required to establish proficiency in single incision laparoscopy. A multicenter analysis revealed a linear improvement in both entry and operating times for SILS cases, with the most substantial decrease (9.2 min to 4.8 min for abdominal entry and 79.4 min to 56.8 min for total operating time) after increasing procedure volume from 10 to 20 cases [6].

Based on available data, outcomes of single incision laparoscopy for minor gynecologic procedures are similar to multiport laparoscopy [1, 2, 4–30].

Abdominal access is often obtained more quickly with single incision laparoscopy, with one study demonstrating a near 50% shorter entry time for SILS. Operating times for adnexal surgery by way of SILS may be increased when compared to multi-port procedures. A meta-analysis of 3 randomized control trials

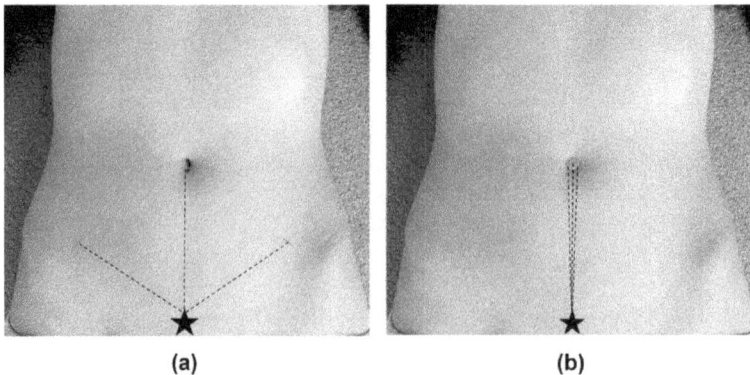

(a)   (b)

Figure 1.
(a) Triangulation in multiport laparoscopy. (b) Loss of triangulation with single incision laparoscopy.

(RCT) published in 2013 demonstrated an increase in operating time of 6.9 minutes for adnexal surgery performed via SILS [8]. A 2017 meta-analysis of 5 RCT found similar increases in operating time [2]. However, subsequent studies not included in these meta-analyses have shown operating time for SILS is not significantly different when compared to multiport laparoscopy[9]. Surgeon proficiency greatly impacts operating time, and has been demonstrated to improve in a linear fashion [6].

Intraoperative complications, such as bowel or vascular injury, blood loss, or conversion to laparotomy are similar. In the 2013 meta-analysis, 2.78% of SILS were converted to multi-port laparoscopy and 0.11% were converted to laparotomy. Of the multi-port laparoscopies, 0.5% were converted to laparotomy. The authors did not distinguish between hysterectomy and adnexal procedures [8]. In the 2017 meta-analysis, no adnexal SILS cases were converted to laparotomy [2]. Decline in hemoglobin on postoperative day 1 was similar in nearly all studies and was found to be statistically similar in the 2016 meta-analysis [4].

Postoperative pain has been found to be comparable in most studies [8–30]. Some have demonstrated less immediate postoperative pain (in recovery and at 6 and 12 hours postoperatively) when a single incision surgical approach is used. Others have also noted less use of postoperative analgesia after SILS. Meta-analyses have demonstrated no significant difference in postoperative pain between the two procedures [2, 4, 9]; however, minor gynecologic surgery, especially adnexal procedures, is generally not associated with a high amount of postoperative pain.

Length of hospital stay is comparable for both types of laparoscopy. Given that the length of the average hospital stay for minor gynecologic surgery is already short, significant improvement is difficult to demonstrate. Resumption of normal postoperative activity is also similar [2, 4, 8].

Patient reported satisfaction with cosmetic results is most often higher with single incision laparoscopy, although some studies have reported no significant difference [8–30]. One analysis conducted by Bush et al. in 2011 revealed that when presented with three illustrations of the placement of port sites - traditional multi-port placement, umbilical SILS, and robotic port placement - over 56% of the 241 female respondents preferred the traditional multiport trocar placement over the SILS (p = .007). Importantly, the illustration of single incision laparoscopy denoted a 2.5 cm umbilical incision that extended past the borders of the model's navel [31] (**Figure 2a**). Many SILS surgeons strive to keep umbilical incisions hidden within the borders of the umbilicus (**Figure 2b**). A similar study conducted in the 1990s - prior to the rise in popularity of laparoscopic gynecology - showed 68% of women

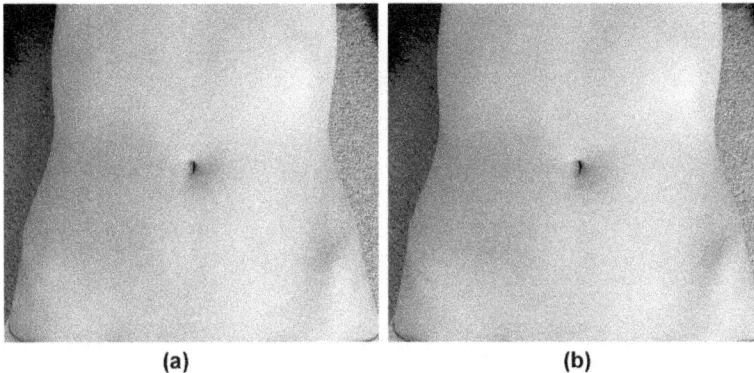

(a)   (b)

Figure 2.
(a) Replication of incision used during Bush study – umbilical incision extends past the umbilicus. (b) Most single incision laparoscopic surgeons will confine the umbilical incision in the borders of the natural orifice.

would choose a Pfannenstiel incision while only 31% would choose multiport laparoscopic incisions, indicating that patient familiarity with the incision type may have played a role in Bush's findings [32].

Data regarding outcomes for single incision non-adnexal surgery is less abundant than that for adnexal procedures. A single RCT with 66 participants undergoing laparoscopic myomectomy by either SILS or multi-port laparoscopy demonstrated no significant differences in surgical outcomes with the exception of more favorable cosmesis and better patient satisfaction in the SILS group [29].

3. Commercially available single incision access systems

A variety of access systems are available for single incision laparoscopic surgery [33, 34] (**Figure 3a-d**). Surgeon preference and comfort level is key when choosing laparoscopic entry. SILS ports were designed to allow the passage of many instruments through one access point with a single, larger skin incision.

3.1 GelPOINT advanced access platform by applied Medical

The GelPOINT system is a gel topped port combined with Alexis wound retractor technology. The Alexis wound retractor provides 360 degree

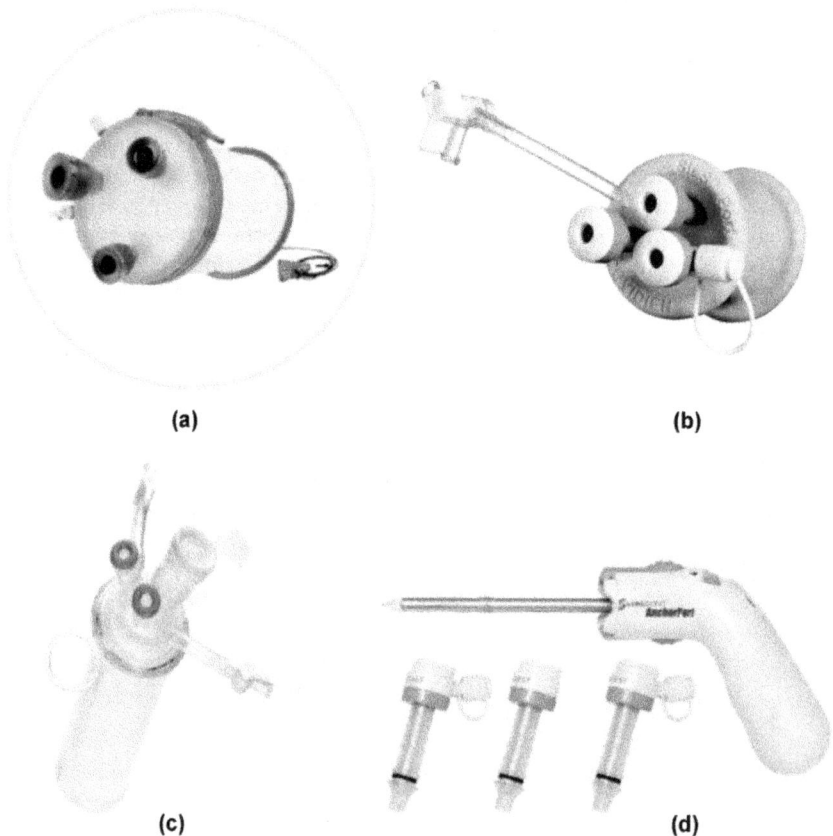

(a)

(b)

(c)

(d)

Figure 3.
(a) GelPOINT system, (b) SILS port, (c) TriPort15, (d) AnchorPort.

retraction of the port site; the rounded retraction allows for better instrument triangulation. Trocars supplied with the device are introduced through the GelSeal cap and may be arranged in any formation. The trocars accommodate instrument diameters from 5 to 12 mm. The device can be used in incisions ranging from 1.5 cm to 7 cm in length. The GelSeal cap has a diameter of 10 cm. The cap can be removed from the Alexis retractor for specimen retrieval [33–35].

The GelPOINT Mini uses the same GelSeal and Alexis retractor technology but with a smaller footprint. This system accommodates incisions up to 4 cm. Triangulation is reduced further with the GelPOINT Mini system, limiting its utility in more complex single incision laparoscopy [35].

3.2 SILS port by Medtronic

The SILS port by Medtronic consists of a blue colored foam, soft, flexible port that maintains pneumoperitoneum by conforming to the body wall. The outer diameter is 49 mm and the inner diameter is 29 mm. The port has an insufflation valve and three instrument placement channels. Three variations of the SILS port are available and can accommodate a range of instrument diameter from 5 mm to 15 mm [33, 34, 36].

3.3 TriPort and QuadPort by advanced surgical concepts

Advanced Surgical Concepts offers three single incision laparoscopy platforms. All three variations are composed of an outer ring connected to an inner ring by a clear retracting sleeve. The distal ring is placed into the abdominal cavity with an introducer which punctures the abdominal wall. After the introducer is removed, the outer ring is passed over the retracting sleeve until it creates a seal. Because of its self adjusting retraction sleeve, this port can be used in abdominal walls up to 10 cm in thickness. The fixed ports are angled in order to minimize instrument crowding. The 10 mm and 15 mm ports are equipped with lip seal valves that allow for the introduction and removal of smaller diameter instruments without losing pneumoperitoneum [33, 34, 37].

One model, the Triport+, contains four instrument ports (three 5 mm and one 10 mm) and two insufflation valves, while Triport15 contains three instrument ports (two 5 mm and one 15 mm) and two insufflation valves. Optimal incision length is between 12 mm and 25 mm. QuadPort contains five instrument ports (two 5 mm, one 10 mm, one 12 mm and one 15 mm) and two insufflation valves. It can be used with incisions 20 mm to 60 mm [37].

3.4 AnchorPort by Conmed

The Anchorport system uses a set of unique self-adjusting, self-anchoring trocars [38]. The 5 mm trocar is available in three lengths: 75 mm, 100 mm, 135 mm. It has a clear bladeless optical tip for direct entry and a pistol-like grip handle. The distal portion of the cannula system adjusts to the patient's abdominal wall thickness with its accordion-like design, which anchors to the body wall for security. The AnchorPort design allows a minimum amount of the cannula tip inside the abdomen; this assists with laparoscopic instrument range of motion and widening instrument angles inside the abdomen. AnchorPort is uniquely designed for single incision laparoscopy; a single skin incision is made and then the trocars are introduced directly into the fascia, maintaining a bridge of tissue between each trocar [33, 34].

4. Accessory products

4.1 Laparoscopes

Traditional lens-based laparoscopes have a rigid shaft and utilize two dimensional views. Laparoscope diameters vary from <1 mm to 15 mm, with the most commonly used diameters being 5 and 10 mm. Classically, laparoscopes utilize charge coupled device (CCD) sensors, in which higher resolution is obtained with larger diameters. In SILS, a smaller diameter, such as 5 mm or less, is often preferred at the expense of resolution in order to maintain maneuverability of surgical instruments [39].

Though flexible tip endoscopy was developed as early as the 1950s, it wasn't until the 2000s that flexible tip laparoscopes with adequate imaging capabilities were developed. The EndoEye Flex video laparoscope with "chip on the tip" design was developed in 2005 by Olympus. It has a deflectable tip that can rotate up to 100 degrees. The latest model allows for high definition video in a 5 mm diameter scope by utilizing complementary metal-oxide semiconductor (CMOS) technology as opposed to CCD. It is also the first autoclavable articulating videoscope, as other designs require chemical sterilization. Stryker has also developed articulating 5 and 10 mm videoscopes, however at the time of this manuscript, the Ideal Eyes HD Articulating Laparoscope does not appear to be available in the current Stryker product catalog. Flexible tip laparoscopes have demonstrated shorter operating times for single incision cholecystectomy, but have not yet been evaluated for gynecologic SILS [39].

Lens angles of rigid laparoscopes can vary. Zero degree scopes are most commonly utilized by gynecologic surgeons in multiport laparoscopy. Angled scopes, however, can be very useful in SILS gynecology by moving the imaging plane out of the line of the operating plane in order to reduce instrument collision. Thirty degree laparoscopes are most commonly used, although 45 degree and 70 degree options are available as well. Variable view laparoscopes developed by Karl Storz allow the surgeon to adjust the lens angle between 0 and 90 degrees without removing the scope from the trocar.

An in-line light cord adapter and low profile camera head are two updates that reduce tangling of cords and instrument collision. Use of a longer laparoscope, as those used in bariatric surgery, may also improve mobility. Future laparoscopes may be cordless and wireless [40].

4.2 Instruments

Traditional laparoscopic instruments are rigid with an average length of 33 cm. Some instruments allow for rotation of the tip while others are fixed. Prebent instruments have been utilized by other specialties in the past but have not been widely utilized in gynecologic SILS [33, 34].

Articulating instruments have been pivotal in improving triangulation constraints of SILS while also increasing the surgeon's range of motion (**Figure 4a and b**). Companies including Medtronic, BD and others manufacture articulating grasping instruments. There are currently 2 articulating 5 mm bipolar instruments on the market. Ethicon's Enseal G2 provides bipolar sealing of vessels up to 7 mm in diameter with 110 degrees of articulation and 360 degree rotation. The Caiman 5 Vessel Sealer by Aesculap offers 80 degrees of articulation, a 26.5 mm sealing length and 23.5 mm cutting length [41, 42].

The ArtiSential line of wristed instruments with 360 degree of freedom was registered with the FDA in 2019. They have yet to be described in single incision gynecology but offer similar range of motion as robotic instruments and may have utility in SILS procedures.

In instances where wider triangulation is necessary, mini laparoscopic instruments can be introduced away from the single incision port site. Many companies promote miniature laparoscopic instruments with diameters 3 mm and under. Some of the smallest diameter instruments are manufactured by Teleflex, which produces instruments with only a 2.4 mm shaft. The instrument is introduced directly through the skin using an integrated needle tip, which eliminates the need for a skin incision or trocar. The product line offers 2 handpieces, 4 types of graspers and 4 monopolar electrosurgical tools.

The magnetically anchored and guidance system (MAGS) was first described in 2007. This device utilizes magnetic coupling of an external handpiece and an internal instrument or camera. The internal components are inserted through a single incision and paired to their external components via magnetic attraction across the

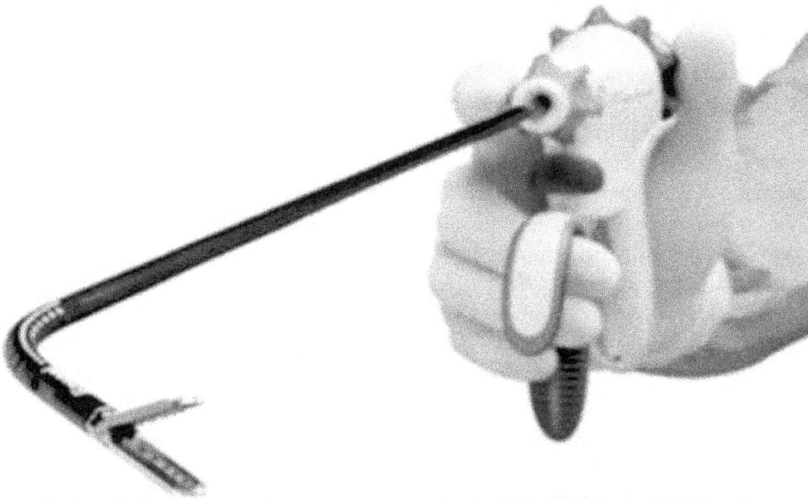

(a)

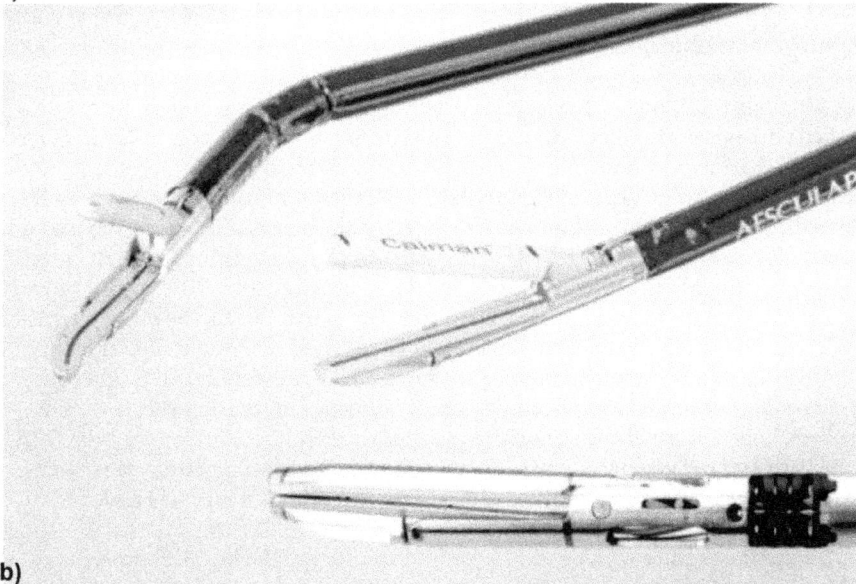

(b)

Figure 4.
Articulating Bipolar Vessel Sealers. (a) Enseal G2, (b) Calman 5.

abdominal wall, up to a maximal thickness of 10 cm. The internal components can then be arranged in an ergonomic configuration by moving the external components along the abdominal wall. MAGS has been utilized in urology and thoracic surgery, but has not yet been seen in gynecologic surgery [43].

4.3 Smoke evacuation systems

The dangers of surgical smoke to the surgical team are well documented. Electrocauterization instruments, lasers, and ultrasonic scalpels all release particulate matter (PM) into the ambient air during both open and laparoscopic surgery. Particles 10 microns or smaller can be inhaled. Studies evaluating the long term effects specific to surgical smoke are insufficient; however the PM found in surgical smoke is associated with coronary artery disease, congestive heart failure, asthma, and chronic obstructive pulmonary disease. Deposits of PM have been found in remote organs, including the brain, and may be associated with increased oxidative stress and systemic inflammation. Long term exposure may be associated with decreased life expectancy [44].

During laparoscopy, surgical smoke also impairs visualization. As simply venting the plume into the ambient air is ill advised, smoke evacuation systems are crucial in providing adequate visualization of structures. Dozens of smoke evacuation systems have been marketed for laparoscopic procedures. ConMed's Airseal, released in 2007, is uniquely beneficial to gynecologic SILS. The Airseal system maintains the pneumoperitoneum, provides constant smoke evacuation and allows valve free port access. The high pressure nozzles of the port's cannula direct recirculated CO_2 gas down into the trocar in order to maintain pressure which creates a horizontal gas barrier across the cannula. Thus, introduction of a smaller caliber instrument or even 2 instruments through a single trocar does not result in loss of pneumoperitoneum. AirSeal has 3 operational modes: AirSeal Mode, Smoke Evacuation Mode, and Standard Insufflation Mode. The system filters particles as small as 0.01 microns [33, 34, 44].

5. Surgical techniques

Although traditionally, the least experienced member of the surgical team is often tasked with uterine manipulation, expert uterine manipulation is often key in gynecologic SILS. Introduction of multiple instruments through a single port site reduces mobility, and manipulation of the uterus can enhance or replace retraction usually done through the abdominal wall. Retroversion of the uterus allows access to the vesicouterine space. Anteversion of the uterus exposes the rectouterine space. Rotational uterine manipulation, rather than straight lateral displacement of the uterus, provides better access to the adnexa of surgical interest. The uterus can also be pushed cephalad to displace the ureters laterally or pulled caudad to access the fundus of a larger uterus.

Creation of a posterior colpotomy during a non-hysterectomy SILS procedure can provide a second point of access for instrumentation, passing suture or removing specimens. Vaginal natural orifice transluminal endoscopic surgery (vNOTES), which utilizes the vaginal as the sole entry point for endoscopic surgery, is discussed in a separate chapter. The techniques described for vNOTES may be employed in complex SILS cases as well.

Temporary sutures can be used to provide retraction during SILS procedures. This technique is often called "puppeteering" [1]. Straight needles are useful in that they can be passed through a trocar or inserted directly through the abdominal wall. Curved needles may be introduced through larger caliber trocars or partially straightened to pass through smaller trocars. Choice of suture is based upon surgeon preference as the suture is removed after the procedure is completed. As long as care is taken to avoid vascular structures, the uterus and adnexa can be retracted with puppet sutures. Large bowel should only be retracted by suturing through the epiploica. Small bowel should not be retracted in this manner due to risk of injury.

Author details

M. Luann Racher* and Ann Marie Mercier
Department of Obstetrics and Gynecology, University of Arkansas for Medical
Sciences, Little Rock, AR, USA

*Address all correspondence to: mlracher@uams.edu

IntechOpen

References

[1] Rao PP, Rao PP, Bhagwat S. Single-incision laparoscopic surgery - current status and controversies. J Minim Access Surg. 2011;7(1):6-16. doi:10.4103/0972-9941.72360

[2] Schmitt A, Crochet P, Knight S, Tourette C, Loundou A, Agostini A. Single-Port Laparoscopy vs Conventional Laparoscopy in Benign Adnexal Diseases: A Systematic Review and Meta-Analysis. J Minim Invasive Gynecol. 2017 Nov-Dec;24(7): 1083-1095. doi: 10.1016/j.jmig.2017. 07.001. Epub 2017 Jul 10. PMID: 28705751.

[3] Supe AN, Kulkarni GV, Supe PA. Ergonomics in laparoscopic surgery. J Minim Access Surg. 2010;6(2):31-36. doi:10.4103/0972-9941.65161

[4] Far SS, Miraj S. Single-incision laparoscopy surgery: a systematic review. *Electron Physician*. 2016;8(10):3088-3095. Published 2016 Oct 25. doi:10.19082/3088

[5] Bradford LS, Boruta DM. Laparoendoscopic single-site surgery in gynecology: a review of the literature, tools, and techniques. Obstet Gynecol Surv. 2013 Apr;68(4):295-304. doi: 10.1097/OGX.0b013e318286f673. PMID: 23943039.

[6] Amanda Nickles Fader, Luis Rojas-Espaillat, Okechukwu Ibeanu, Francis C. Grumbine, Pedro F. Escobar, Laparoendoscopic single-site surgery (LESS) in gynecology: a multi-institutional evaluation, American Journal of Obstetrics and Gynecology, Volume 203, Issue 5, 2010, Pages 501. e1-501.e6

[7] Zhao M, Zhao J, Hua K, Zhu Z, Hu C. Single-incision multiport laparoscopy versus multichannel-tipped single port laparoscopy in gynecologic surgery: outcomes and benefits. Int J Clin Exp Med. 2015 Sep 15;8(9):14992-14998. PMID: 26628982; PMCID: PMC4658871.

[8] Murji A, Patel VI, Leyland N, Choi M. Single-incision laparoscopy in gynecologic surgery: a systematic review and meta-analysis. Obstet Gynecol. 2013 Apr;121(4):819-828. doi: 10.1097/AOG.0b013e318288828c. PMID: 23635683.

[9] Karasu Y, Akselim B, Kavak Cömert D, Ergün Y, Ülker K. Comparison of single-incision and conventional laparoscopic surgery for benign adnexal masses. Minim Invasive Ther Allied Technol. 2017 Oct;26(5):278-283. doi: 10.1080/ 13645706.2017.1299763. Epub 2017 Mar 14. PMID: 28290726.

[10] Cho YJ, Kim ML, Lee SY, Lee HS, Kim JM, Joo KY. Laparoendoscopic single-site surgery (LESS) versus conventional laparoscopic surgery for adnexal preservation: a randomized controlled study. Int J Womens Health. 2012;4:85-91. doi: 10.2147/ijwh.s29761. Epub 2012 Mar 13. PMID: 22448110; PMCID: PMC3310352.

[11] Hoyer-Sørensen C., Vistad I., and Ballard K.: Is single-port laparoscopy for benign adnexal disease less painful than conventional laparoscopy? A single-center randomized controlled trial. Fertil Steril 2012; 98: pp. 973-979

[12] Fagotti A., Bottoni C., Vizzielli G., et al: Postoperative pain after conventional laparoscopy and laparoendoscopic single site surgery (LESS) for benign adnexal disease: a randomized trial. Fertil Steril 2011; 96: pp. 255-259

[13] Im K.S., Koo Y.J., Kim J.B., and Kwon Y.S.: Laparoendoscopic single-site surgery versus conventional laparoscopic surgery for adnexal tumors: a comparison of surgical

outcomes and postoperative pain outcomes. Kaohsiung J Med Sci 2011; 27: pp. 91-95

[14] Yoo E.H., and Shim E.: Single-port access compared with three-port laparoscopic adnexal surgery in a randomized controlled trial. J Int Med Res 2013; 41: pp. 673-680

[15] Yoon B.S., Kim Y.S., Seong S.J., et al: Impact on ovarian reserve after laparoscopic ovarian cystectomy with reduced port number: a randomized controlled trial. Eur J Obstet Gynecol Reprod Biol 2014; 176: pp. 34-38

[16] Kim T.J., Lee Y.Y., An J.J., et al: Does single-port access (SPA) laparoscopy mean reduced pain? A retrospective cohort analysis between SPA and conventional laparoscopy. Eur J Obstet Gynecol Reprod Biol 2012; 162: pp. 71-74

[17] Lee Y.Y., Kim T.J., Kim C.J., et al: Single port access laparoscopic adnexal surgery versus conventional laparoscopic adnexal surgery: a comparison of peri-operative outcomes. Eur J Obstet Gynecol Reprod Biol 2010; 151: pp. 181-184

[18] Buda A., Cuzzocrea M., Montanelli L., et al: Evaluation of patient satisfaction using the EORTC IN-PATSAT32 questionnaire and surgical outcome in single-port surgery for benign adnexal disease: observational comparison with traditional laparoscopy. Diagn Ther Endosc 2013; 2013: pp. 578392

[19] Park J.Y., Kim D.Y., Kim S.H., Suh D.S., Kim J.H., and Nam J.H.: Laparoendoscopic single-site compared with conventional laparoscopic ovarian cystectomy for ovarian endometrioma. J Minim Invasive Gynecol 2015; 22: pp. 813-819

[20] Lee I.O., Yoon J.W., Chung D., et al: A comparison of clinical and surgical outcomes between laparo-endoscopic single-site surgery and traditional multiport laparoscopic surgery for adnexal tumors. Obstet Gynecol Sci 2014; 57: pp. 386-392

[21] Kim M.L., Song T., Seong S.J., et al: Comparison of single-port, two-port and four-port laparoscopic surgery for cyst enucleation in benign ovarian cysts. Gynecol Obstet Invest 2013; 76: pp. 57-63

[22] Bedaiwy M.A., Starks D., Hurd W., and Escobar P.F.: Laparoendoscopic single-site surgery in patients with benign adnexal disease: a comparative study. Gynecol Obstet Invest 2012; 73: pp. 294-298

[23] Bedaiwy M.A., Sheyn D., Eghdami L., et al: Laparoendoscopic single-site surgery for benign ovarian cystectomies. Gynecol Obstet Invest 2015; 79: pp. 179-183

[24] Yim G.W., Lee M., Nam E.J., Kim S., Kim Y.T., and Kim S.W.: Is single-port access laparoscopy less painful than conventional laparoscopy for adnexal surgery? A comparison of postoperative pain and surgical outcomes. Surg Innov 2013; 20: pp. 46-54

[25] Huang B.S., Wang P.H., Tsai H.W., Hsu T.F., Yen M.S., and Chen Y.J.: Single-port compared with conventional laparoscopic cystectomyfor ovarian dermoid cysts. Taiwan J Obstet Gynecol 2014; 53: pp. 523-529

[26] Liliana M, Alessandro P, Giada C, Luca M. Single-port access laparoscopic hysterectomy: a new dimension of minimally invasive surgery. J Gynecol Endosc Surg. 2011;2(1):11-17. doi:10.4103/0974-1216.85273

[27] Kim SK, Lee JH, Lee JR, Suh CS, Kim SH. Laparoendoscopic single-site myomectomy versus conventional laparoscopic myomectomy: a comparison of surgical outcomes.

J Minim Invasive Gynecol. 2014 Sep-Oct;21(5):775-781. doi: 10.1016/j.jmig.2014.03.002. Epub 2014 Mar 12. PMID: 24632396.

[28] Choi CH, Kim TH, Kim SH, Choi JK, Park JY, Yoon A, Lee YY, Kim TJ, Lee JW, Kim BG, Bae DS. Surgical outcomes of a new approach to laparoscopic myomectomy: single-port and modified suture technique. J Minim Invasive Gynecol. 2014 Jul-Aug;21(4):580-585. doi: 10.1016/j.jmig.2013.12.096. Epub 2013 Dec 31. PMID: 24384072.

[29] Lee D, Kim SK, Kim K, Lee JR, Suh CS, Kim SH. Advantages of Single-Port Laparoscopic Myomectomy Compared with Conventional Laparoscopic Myomectomy: A Randomized Controlled Study. J Minim Invasive Gynecol. 2018 Jan;25(1):124-132. doi: 10.1016/j.jmig.2017.08.651. Epub 2017 Aug 18. PMID: 28826957.

[30] Ramesh B, Vidyashankar M, Bharathi B. Single incision laparoscopic myomectomy. J Gynecol Endosc Surg. 2011;2(1):61-63. doi:10.4103/0974-1216.85288

[31] Bush AJ, Morris SN, Millham FH, et al. Women's preference for minimally invasive incisions. J Minim Invasive Gynecol. 2011; 18: 640-643

[32] Currie I., Onwude J.L., Jarvis G.J.: A comparative study of the cosmetic appeal of abdominal incisions used for hysterectomy. Br J Obstet Gynaecol 1996; 103: pp. 252-254.

[33] Romanelli, J.R., Earle, D.B. Single-port laparoscopic surgery: an overview. Surg Endosc **23**, 1419-1427 (2009).

[34] Kumar, Chigurupathi Venkata Pavan. "Different types of single incision laparoscopy surgery (SILS) ports." *World J Laparosc Surg* 4.1 (2011): 47-51.

[35] Applied Medical. GelPOINT Advanced Access Platforms. 2019

[36] Medtronic. Laparoscopic Access Catalogue. June 2020

[37] Advanced Surgical Concepts. Laparoendoscopic Single Site Surgery Access Devices. 2020.

[38] ConMed. Advanced Surgical Product Catalog. 2019.

[39] Matsui Y, Ryota H, Sakaguchi T, Nakatani K, Matsushima H, Yamaki S, Hirooka S, Yamamoto T, Kwon AH. Comparison of a flexible-tip laparoscope with a rigid straight laparoscope for single-incision laparoscopic cholecystectomy. Am Surg. 2014 Dec;80(12):1245-1249. PMID: 25513924.

[40] Chatzipapas, Ioannis PhD; Kathopoulis, Nikolaos MD; Siemou, Panagiota PhD; Protopapas, Athanasios PhD Wireless Laparoscopy in the 2020s, Obstetrics & Gynecology: November 2020 - Volume 136 - Issue 5 - p 908-911

[41] Ethicon. Enseal G2 Articulating Tissue Sealer Brochure. 2020.

[42] Aesculap. Caiman Vessel Sealers. March 2019.

[43] Best SL, Cadeddu JA. Development of magnetic anchoring and guidance systems for minimally invasive surgery. Indian J Urol. 2010;26(3):418-422. doi:10.4103/0970-1591.70585

[44] Limchantra IV, Fong Y, Melstrom KA. Surgical Smoke Exposure in Operating Room Personnel: A Review. JAMA Surg. 2019;154(10):960-967. doi:10.1001/jamasurg.2019.2515

Chapter 2

Fundamentals of the Robotic Assisted Laparoscopic Single Port System and Utility in Minor Gynecologic Surgery

John R. Wagner

Abstract

This chapter will introduce the single port robotic system. Topics include an introduction to the robotic single site port, the trocars, and the single site instruments. Step-by-step instruction is provided on how to create the umbilical incision and properly insert the single site port and trocars. The advantages and disadvantages of single port robotic surgery compared to multiple port robotic surgery and laparoscopic single site surgery are reviewed. Surgical tips and tricks are provided throughout each section to maximize efficiency, minimize complications, and overcome inherent limitations of the robotic single site system. The utility of the robotic single site platform for performing minor gynecologic surgery is discussed. Finally, a simple method for umbilical closure is described.

Keywords: robotic assisted laparoscopic, gynecologic surgery, umbilical incision, umbilical closure

1. Introduction

This chapter will introduce the single port robotic system. Topics include an introduction to the robotic single site port, the trocars, and the single site instruments. Step-by-step instruction is provided on how to create the umbilical incision and properly insert the single site port and trocars. The advantages and disadvantages of single port robotic surgery compared to multiple port robotic surgery and laparoscopic single site surgery are reviewed. Surgical tips and tricks are provided throughout each section to maximize efficiency, minimize complications, and overcome the inherent limitations of the robotic single site system. The utility of the robotic single site platform for performing minor gynecologic surgery is discussed in detail. Finally, a simple method for umbilical closure is described.

2. Advantages of robotic single site surgery

Single site surgery, whether laparoscopic or robotic, offers several advantages over traditional multiple port surgery. The anatomy of the umbilicus is unique. It is the only part of the anterior abdominal wall where the skin and peritoneum are located directly adjacent to each other, without intervening fat and muscle. As a result, the umbilicus provides easy access to the abdomen, even in morbidly obese patients. Furthermore, the stalk of the umbilicus is composed primarily of fibrotic scar tissue with minimal vascularity. Consequently, most umbilical incisions are relatively bloodless [1]. In addition, single site surgery obviously eliminates the risks associated with the placement of accessory trocars, including bleeding, flank hematomas, incisional hernias, and visceral injury. The lack of additional trocars also contributes to less post-operative pain [2, 3].

The most obvious advantage of single site surgery, however, is cosmesis. Even a 2-3 cm incision can be hidden in the umbilicus, and it often becomes virtually invisible as it heals [4]. The poor vascularity of the umbilicus also minimizes the risk for a postoperative hematoma and virtually eliminates the risk for keloid formation [5].

The most functional advantage of single site surgery is using the umbilical incision for specimen retrieval. The lack of intervening muscle and fat provides easy access to the surgical specimen. Specimen retrieval is easy, and any morcellation required is readily accomplished by bringing the specimen bag up through the umbilical incision [6].

Robotic single site surgery offers advantages over traditional laparoscopic single site surgery. The 3-D binocular vision provided by the robotic platform allows for better depth perception and facilitates more precise surgical movements. Although the only wristed instrument is the robotic needle driver, this is also a significant advantage over all "straight stick" laparoscopic instruments. The binocular vision and wristed needle driver greatly facilitate intracorporeal suturing and knot tying. The needle driver can also be employed as a grasper and its dexterity can improve exposure for adhesiolysis or facilitate the excision of an ovarian cyst. Finally, the robotic single site platform is more ergonomic and intuitive. Intra-abdominally, the surgeon's right hand controls the right sided instrument and the left hand controls

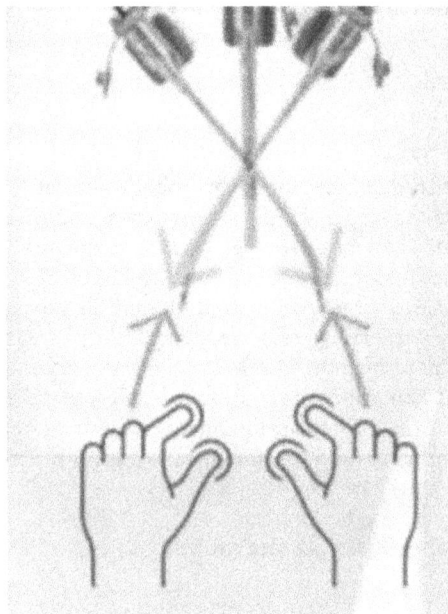

Figure 1.
Surgeon's right hand controls the right instrument intra abdominally and vice versa.

the left-sided instrument, even though, externally, these instruments and trocars are located on the opposite side (**Figure 1**).

3. Disadvantages of robotic single site surgery

Compared to traditional multiple port robotic surgery, there are some disadvantages to the single site robotic system. The robotic single site instruments are relatively primitive. There are no advanced energy instruments such as the harmonic scalpel or bipolar transection tools built into the robotic single site system. The only unipolar tool available is the hook; the scissors do not have any unipolar power capability. In addition, the required semi-rigid flexibility of the robotic single site instruments leads to a relatively weak grasping force. This is most readily apparent when attempting to suture with the needle driver or when trying to hold tissue on tension. Furthermore, even though the needle driver is wristed, it has less range of motion than traditional robotic instruments.

Finally, the "working space" of the robotic single site system is limited compared to traditional robotic surgery. The trocar length is fixed, and the instruments cannot be retracted back any further than the tip of the trocars. This can make surgery more difficult in the setting of big pathology such as a large fibroid uterus or large ovarian cyst. In addition, in patients of short stature, the distance from the umbilicus to the pelvis is often smaller, and this can further compromise the functional workspace.

Access by the assistant surgeon can be compromised with the robotic single site system. Lateral movements can lead to repeated collisions (often coined "sword fighting") between the instruments and camera both inside the abdomen and outside. The most unencumbered instrument movements by the assistant are those performed in an anterior to posterior direction — parallel to the camera. Despite these disadvantages, the robotic single site system can readily handle most gynecologic surgery. Various techniques for overcoming these disadvantages are discussed in the "Tips and Tricks" section of this chapter.

4. Abdominal entry

The initial step in any single site operation, whether robotic or laparoscopic, is the umbilical incision. Various incisions have been proposed, but the simplest, easiest, and most cosmetic approach is a midline vertical incision right through the center of the umbilicus. Local anesthesia (with or without epinephrine) is injected into the base of the umbilicus. Toothed forceps placed at the superior and inferior edges of the umbilicus are used to elevate the skin and an incision is made vertically through the center of the umbilicus. Allis clamps are then placed laterally and used to elevate the skin edges. With the edges elevated, the stalk of the umbilicus is palpated as a horizontal band of fascia in the center of the incision. Kocher clamps are then placed laterally on this fascia band, and the Allis clamps are removed. While elevating with the Kocher clamps, an incision is then made vertically in the fascia. The fascial incision is then sharply enlarged to allow the surgeon to bluntly enter the abdomen digitally. The skin and fascial incisions are then enlarged as needed. For robotic single site surgery, a 2-3 cm incision is required. This is slightly larger than what may be required for laparoscopic single site surgery, depending on the intended operation. The fascial incision should be extended vertically in both directions until it is slightly larger than the skin incision (**Figures 2–5**).

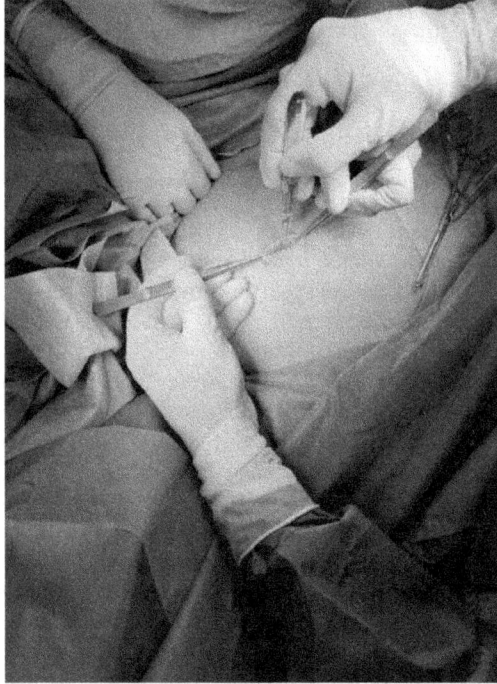

Figure 2.
Vertical umbilical skin incision.

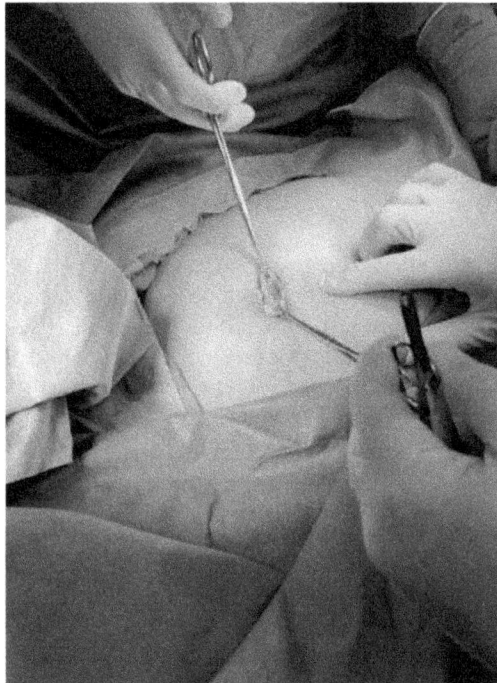

Figure 3.
Allis clamps placed bilaterally on the skin edges and gently elevated.

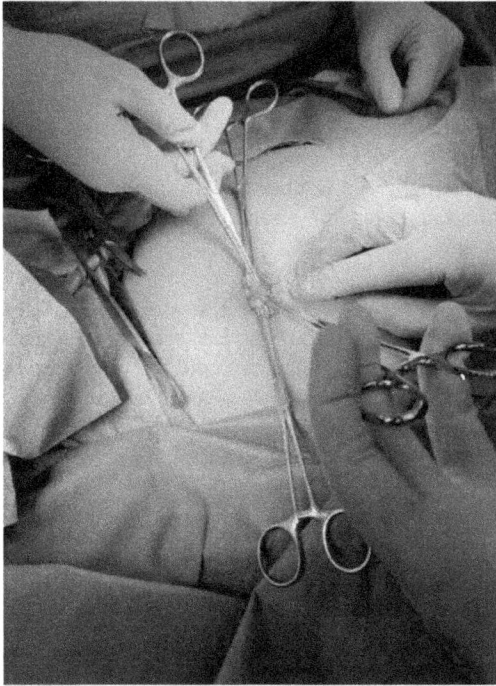

Figure 4.
Kocher clamps placed bilaterally on the umbilical stalk which appears as a horizontal fascial band in the incision.

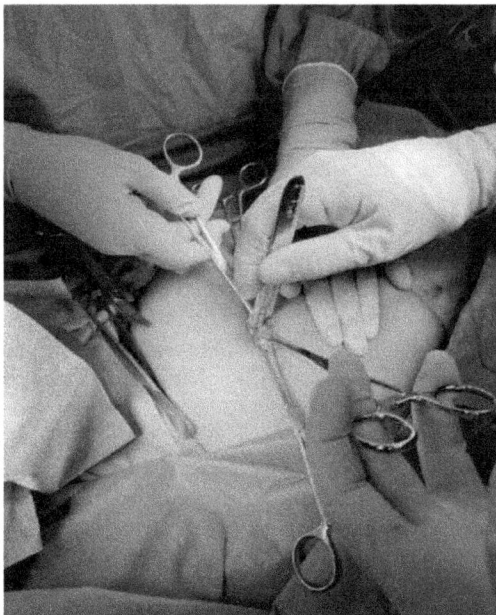

Figure 5.
Vertical fascial skin incision followed by blunt digital abdominal entry.

4.1 Tips and tricks

1. Aggressive incisions in the skin and fascia facilitate entry, and hesitant incisions complicate entry. The base and stalk of the umbilicus is composed of thick fibrotic scar tissue, thicker than any other part of the anterior abdominal wall. A number 15 scalpel is used, as bigger blades may not reach the base of the umbilicus, especially if it is anatomically smaller. Generally, the entire length of the number 15 blade is needed to achieve proper incision depth in both the skin and fascia.

2. Not infrequently a hernia is encountered in the umbilicus during initial entry. Virtually all of these are fat containing. Excision of any excess fat with unipolar cautery easily restores normal anatomy, and the operation then continues as planned. When an umbilical hernia is encountered upon entry, closure of the umbilicus at the end of surgery is done with either a permanent suture such as 0-Prolene or a significantly delayed absorbable suture such as 0-PDS.

3. Patients with a previous umbilical hernia repair require special attention. If mesh present, entry is accomplished by making an incision through the mesh just as it is performed for the fascial incision. During closure, the mesh is re-approximated with a permanent suture such as 0-Prolene

4. Periumbilical adhesions can also complicate surgical entry. When these are encountered, the fascia is elevated with Kocher clamps and the adhesions are lysed sharply under direct visualization as far as possible. Insertion of a laparoscopic single site port with a small intra-abdominal footprint (such as the Covidien SILS port or the Gel-Point Mini) then allows for further adhesiolysis laparoscopically under direct visualization. Once the adhesions are taken down, the robotic single site port can then be inserted without difficulty in the usual manner

5. The robotic single site system

The single site robotic system consists of three main components — the port, the individual instruments, and the various trocars.

5.1 The single site port

The robotic port is a flexible hourglass shaped device designed to sit in the umbilicus. It has a lip on each end. The inner lip is designed to sit in the peritoneal cavity and the outer lip above the skin. The port itself has four lumens for the various single site trocars and an insufflation channel with a plastic trocar embedded in it. An arrow is present on the exposed lip and the port should be oriented so that this arrow points towards the intended operative field. The two channels closest to the operative field are for the camera trocar and the assistant trocar (**Figures 6** and 7). The two port channels furthest away for the operative field (or more cephalad in the case of gynecologic surgery) are for the single site trocars.

In preparation for port insertion, place a Kocher clamp laterally on each side of the incision, holding both the peritoneum and the fascia together. Lifting these clamps provides counter traction to facilitate port insertion and holding both the peritoneum and the fascia together prevents pre-peritoneal insertion of the port. Some surgeons alternatively prefer to use "S" shaped retractors to elevate the

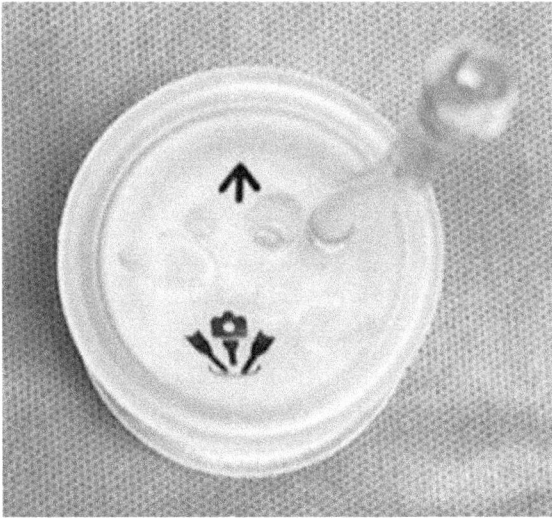

Figure 6.
Robotic port.

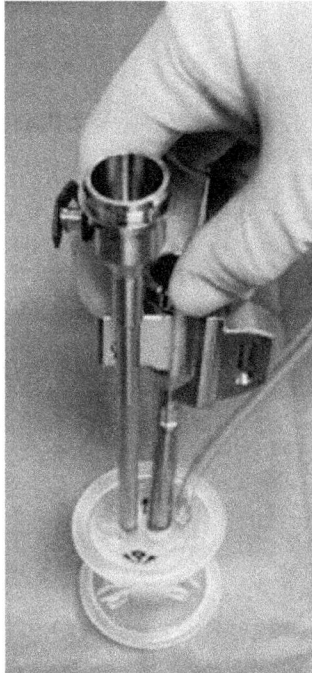

Figure 7.
Robotic port with the camera trocar and assistant trocar in place.

anterior abdominal wall instead of Kocher clamps; however, I have found this method less effective. Two long Kelly clamps are then placed on the port as shown (**Figure 7**). With the surgeon's non-dominant hand steadying the port, the dominant hand holds the inferiorly placed Kelly clamp and inserts the port into the

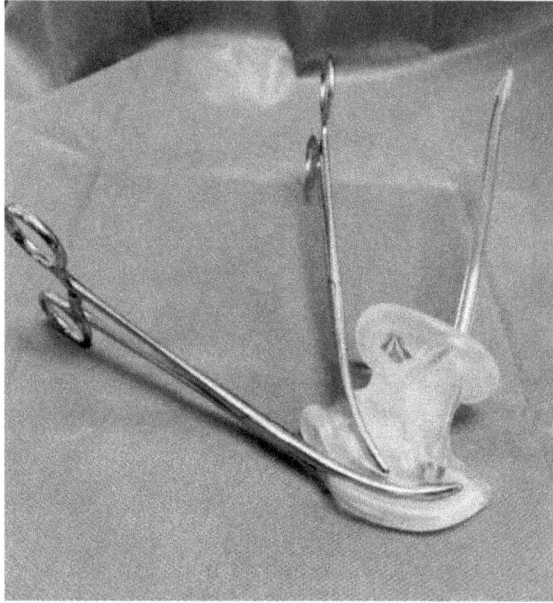

Figure 8.
Kocher clamps placed on robotic port to facilitate placement.

abdomen with a "C" shaped motion. It is important to assure that the leading edge of the port is in the abdominal cavity at this time. While applying constant pressure to hold the port in place with the surgeon's non-dominant hand, the dominant hand then removes the inferior Kelly clamp and grabs the superior one. Final insertion of the port is then accomplished by pushing the second clamp in a vertical direction, essentially dragging the port into the umbilicus (**Figure 8A and B**). During insertion of the port, the assistant provides constant counter traction by elevating the anterior abdominal wall with the Kocher clamps. Once the port is in the umbilicus, the second clamp is then removed. Before the Kocher clamps are removed, digital pressure is applied to the center of the port to push the port as deeply into the umbilicus as possible. When properly placed, the inner lip of the port should be located in the abdominal cavity and the outer lip above the level of the skin. The port is then adjusted so that the arrow is pointed towards the operative field. This assures that, when the single site trocars are placed, they will be properly oriented to the surgical field. At this point the abdomen is inflated and the patient is placed in the Trendelenburg position.

5.2 Tips and tricks

1. Initial placement of the robotic port can be a challenge when the umbilicus is relatively deep, as it can be difficult to place the inner lip of the port past the peritoneum. To overcome this, it helps to place an extra small Alexis retractor in the umbilicus. Once the Alexis retractor is folded down, the depth of the umbilicus is reduced, and the peritoneum is pulled upward towards the skin. Using two Kocher clamps to elevate the fascia bilaterally, the robotic port can then be placed in the umbilicus inside the Alexis retractor. Some surgeons routinely use this technique to place the robotic single incision port (**Figures 9 and 10**).

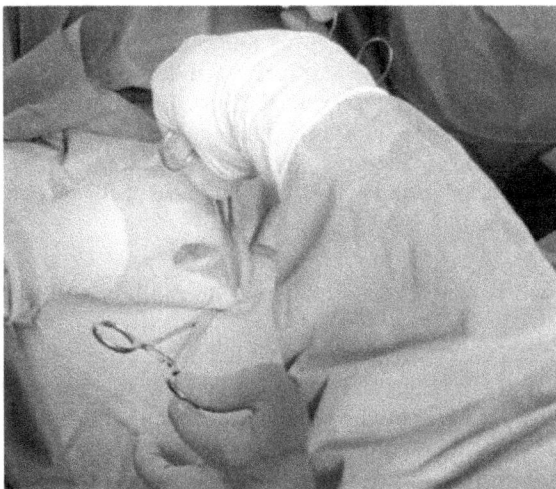

Figure 9.
Initial Kocher clamp slides the robotic port into the abdomen in a "C" shaped motion.

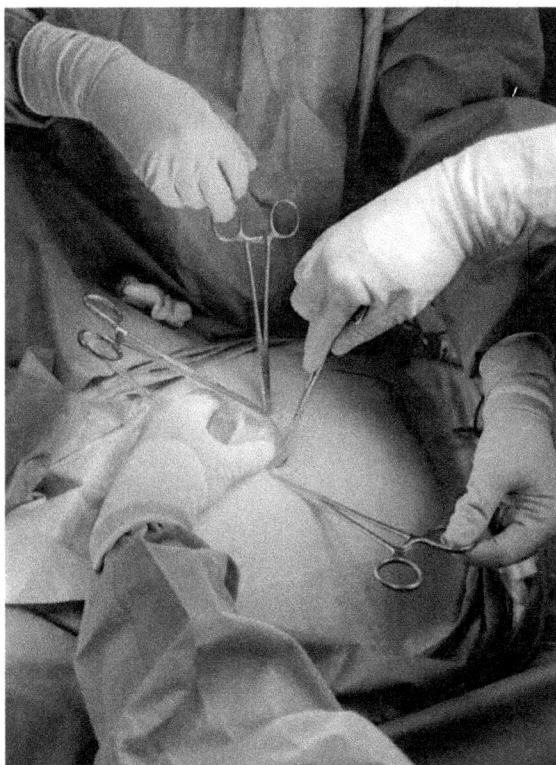

Figure 10.
Second Kocher clamp drags the port completely into the umbilicus after removing the first clamp.

2. The robotic single site port is relatively fragile. Excessive force will cause it to tear which can lead to difficulty maintaining an adequate pneumoperitoneum during surgery. If difficulty is encountered with insertion, enlarge the skin and fascial incisions by a millimeter or two and re-attempt port placement.

3. The key to easy port placement is to make sure that the tip of the second Kelly clamp is intra-peritoneal once the first Kelly clamp is removed. This allows the second Kelly clamp to pull the port into the abdomen rather than to push it in. Pushing it in often leads to tearing of the port. To maintain the proper location of the second Kelly clamp while removing the first one, the operator's non-dominant hand needs to maintain firm and constant pressure holding the port in place. If the port slips out even slightly, the tip of the second Kelly will not be intraperitoneal.

6. The trocars

The camera trocar is straight and 8 mm in diameter. It is placed through the vertical middle channel between the plastic insufflation tube and the assistant trocar channel. The assistant trocars are also straight and either 5 mm or 10 mm in diameter. Either one can be placed through the vertical assistant channel adjacent to the camera trocar. The 5 mm single site trocars are curved and come in two sizes — one shorter and one longer. They are placed through the remaining channels on the robotic port. These channels traverse the port diagonally, so that the right trocar emerges one the left side intra-abdominally, and vice versa. Once placed, the trocars criss cross each other in the port (**Figure 11**). All trocars are inserted until the thin black line on the trocars reaches the external edge of the port. All of the trocars have a blunt obturator to assist with insertion through the robotic port.

The trocars are inserted after the robotic port has been placed in the umbilicus, the abdomen insufflated, and the patient placed in Trendelenburg position. The

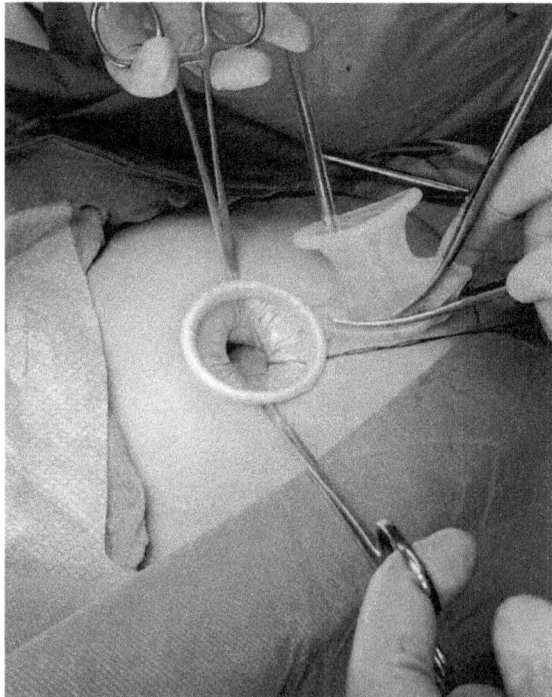

Figure 11.
With the Alexis retractor secured to the umbilicus, and Kocher clamps attached to the fascia, the robotic port is inserted in the usual manner.

camera trocar is introduced first. With the surgeon and assistant stabilizing the robotic port in the umbilicus, the trocar is placed through the appropriate channel in a direction parallel to the long axis of the port. Unlike multi-port robotic surgery, the robot is docked at this point, the camera trocar is attached to the appropriate robotic arm, and targeting is performed. Docking at this stage facilitates placement of the additional trocars.

To place the 5 mm curved single site trocars, the laparoscope is placed in the 30 degree up position and oriented 90 degrees from the pelvis towards the right lower quadrant of the abdomen. The intra-abdominal right sided trocar is placed first (from the left side of the patient). Using one hand to stabilize the port, the surgeon's other hand inserts the trocar through the port in a direction perpendicular to the long axis of the patient, from left to right. Once through the port and within the abdomen, the laparoscope can then visualize the tip of the trocar with the obturator in it. Under continuous laparoscopic visualization, the 5 mm trocar is then turned and advanced towards the pelvis until the thin black line on the trocar shaft reaches the robotic port. After placing the left-sided trocar into the right intra-abdominal space, the laparoscope is turned 180 degrees and oriented to visualize the left lower quadrant of the abdomen. The right-sided trocar is then placed into the left lower abdominal region using the same technique. The robotic arms are then docked to the curved trocars. Keeping the laparoscope in the 30 degree up position the assistant trocar is then placed parallel to the camera trocar.

6.1 Tips and tricks

1. Lubricating the trocars makes insertion easier. Surgilube lubricating jelly helps. However, in my experience, coating the trocars and obturator tip with a little blood and grease from the umbilical incision works best and makes trocar insertion very smooth.

2. When attaching the robotic arms to the trocars, it helps to visualize the operative field with both trocars visible on the monitor. This orients the trocars for easy docking.

7. The instruments

The robotic single site instruments are all 5 mm, semi-rigid, and flexible. The semi-rigid nature of the instruments allows them to effectively manipulate tissue. The flexibility allows them to be inserted through the curved single site trocars. However, that flexibility comes at a price — the grasping power of the instruments is significantly weaker than standard robotic instruments. This makes it harder to hold tissue on tension, and it makes needles in the needle driver more likely to pivot with any lateral tension. Another drawback is that the only instruments with electrical energy are the unipolar hook and the bipolar forceps. The scissors have no electrical power. The robotic single site instruments currently available are

- 5 mm Maryland Dissector

- 5 mm Hem-o-Lok ML Clip Applier

- 5 mm Suction Irrigator

- 5 mm Cadiere Grasper

- 5 mm Curved Scissors

- 5 mm Fundus Grasper

- 5 mm Crocodile Grasper

- 5 mm Maryland Bipolar Forceps

- 5 mm Curved Needle Driver

- 5 mm Permanent Cautery Hook

- 5 mm Fenestrated Bipolar Forceps

- 5 mm Wristed Needle Driver

While this appears to be a wide array of instruments, in reality, most single site surgery is performed primarily with the bipolar forceps, unipolar hook, and wristed needle driver. The bipolar forceps functions as a grasper. As a result, unless extra tension is needed for traction, most of the other graspers will be used infrequently. Without unipolar power, the scissors become less valuable. The scissors are probably most useful only when operating near bowel or other situations where unipolar energy may pose an unnecessary risk.

The unipolar hook is an instrument relatively unfamiliar to gynecologic surgeons. As a result, there is a learning curve associated with its use. However, most experienced surgeons readily adapt to it without much difficulty.

7.1 Tips and tricks

1. When transecting tissue with the hook, constant tension is required. Otherwise, the hook will tend to over-cauterize the tissue and stick to it. This not only makes the surgery look awkward but tends to cause bleeding from the tissue when the hook is pulled free.

8. General tips and tricks

As discussed previously, there are some inherent disadvantages in the robotic single site system. The purpose of this section is to offer some practical advice to help overcome these limitations

1. Performing surgery with the robotic laparoscope in the 30 degree up position (as opposed not 30 degree down) dramatically increases the ability of the surgical assistant to aid in the operation. Thirty degree up places the robotic laparoscope in a more vertical position. This provides easy access to the abdominal cavity via the assistant trocar. In this position, when the assistant places an instrument, it presents to the surgeon right between the single site trocars in the middle of the operative field. The major advantage of this positioning is that it allows introduction of advanced energy into the operative field in a functional manner (**Figure 12**).

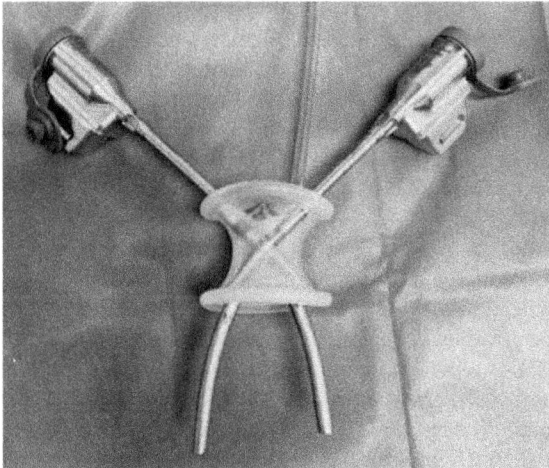

Figure 12.
Single site trocars cross within the robotic port.

2. For instance, when performing a single site hysterectomy, I routinely utilize the 30 degree up positioning for most of the surgery. After isolating the uterine vessels, I grasp them with the single site instruments distally and proximally. My assistant can then easily secure the pedicle with a Ligasure device brought through the assistant trocar. The 30 degree up positioning also allows more freedom of movement for the assistant to manipulate tissue laterally and assist the surgeon.

3. The most obvious tip for facilitating the performance of single site robotic surgery is to add an 8 mm accessory robotic trocar laterally to the umbilicus. The colloquial term for this would be "single site plus one." A right-handed surgeon would likely place this on the patient's right side; the opposite placement is preferred for left-handed surgeons. All regular wristed robotic instruments are then potentially available to be placed through this port, including the Vessel Sealer, unipolar scissors, single tooth tenaculum, or needle drivers with (more wristing capability and more grasping power). Adding an 8 mm plus one port is a great way to get started with single site surgery.

4. Despite the fact that most single-site robotic gynecologic surgery is performed with the shorter curved trocars, one of the biggest difficulties to contend with is that the workspace is still limited. The trocars are fixed in length, and the instruments cannot be retracted back past the trocar tips. However, this limitation can be overcome with several strategies. First, it helps to pull the tissue to be operated on into the pelvis. This is somewhat counter-intuitive to the normal pelvic surgeon. In general, we tend to elevate tissue or push the pelvic organs cephalad with a vaginal manipulator. Retracting the tissue inferiorly pulls it into the workspace of the single site instruments. Second, a small advantage can be gained by pulling the single site trocars back slightly so that the black line on the trocar is 1-2 cm above the robotic port. This technique can be helpful with larger pathology or if access is needed to the pelvic brim or sacral promontory.

5. Passing sutures and needles can only be done through the 10 mm assistant trocar. 10 mm needles tend to easily pass into the abdomen through the port.

However, retrieval can be difficult and frustrating. Often the needle can get caught in the trocar tip, become dislodged from the grasper holding it, and fall back into the abdominal cavity. One solution is to anchor the used needles into the peritoneum in the midline of the anterior abdominal wall. Multiple needles can be stored in this manner, When the procedure is completed, the needles can be placed in a laparoscopic bag. Once the robotic port is removed, the bag can be retrieved through the umbilicus with the needles in it.

6. Make the umbilical incision as small as possible to allow placement of the robotic port. Too large an incision increases the risk for air leakage around the port and can lead to difficulty maintaining an adequate pneumoperitoneum during surgery. When creating the incision, keep in mind that it can always be made bigger, but it cannot be made smaller. If a 10 mm assistant trocar is not needed during the surgery, an 8 mm AirSeal trocar with a 5 mm channel (specifically made for robotic single site surgery) can be inserted through the robotic port. The AirSeal trocar will maintain the pneumoperitoneum even with significant leakage of gas.

7. When operating laterally the workspace can also be limited. Angling the camera way from the horizontal axis towards the lateral pelvis can overcome the obstacle. When the camera is angled, it allows for greater lateral movement of the single site instruments. Such a strategy helps access areas such as the pelvic brim or the base of the infundibulopelvic ligament.

8. Cauterizing a vascular pedicle such as the infundibulopelvic ligament can take longer due to the weaker grasping power of the bipolar forceps. When bipolar cautery is engaged, bubbling can be seen around the forceps. The pedicle is adequately cauterized when the bubbling recedes. Cautery should continue until this is seen, and only then should the pedicle be cut.

9. Most gynecologic surgery is performed using the shorter 5 mm curved trocars. However, the longer trocars can assist with suturing deep in the pelvis, particularly the vaginal cuff. The semi-rigid nature of the single site instruments can make it difficult to drive a needle through relatively tough tissue. The instruments tend to bend when tension is applied, and this weakens the force that can be applied to the needle in order to drive it through tissue. Exchanging the shorter 5 mm trocar for the longer one minimizes the bending of the needle driver when force is applied. This increases the driving force that can be applied to the needle to drive it through tissue.

9. Closure of the umbilicus

Once the port is removed, the fascia and peritoneum are closed with a single running non-locking 0 Vicryl suture. With the fascia closed, flaps are created bilaterally by undermining the skin on either side of the incision until all tension is released. This assures that the umbilicus will appear symmetric when finally closed. Several millimeters of skin are then trimmed on either side along the entire length of the vertical incision. More skin is trimmed from the center of the incision and less inferiorly or superiorly. Trimming of the skin improves blood flow to the edges. Given the generally poor blood flow to the umbilicus, freshening the edges improves healing. Additionally, trimming the skin makes the size of the incision smaller when it is ultimately closed; it tends to pull the incision into the umbilicus.

The base of the umbilicus is then recreated. One or two 2–0 Vicryl sutures on a non-cutting needle are then used to tack the middle of each half of the incision to the fascia. A non-cutting needle is used to avoid inadvertently cutting the fascial

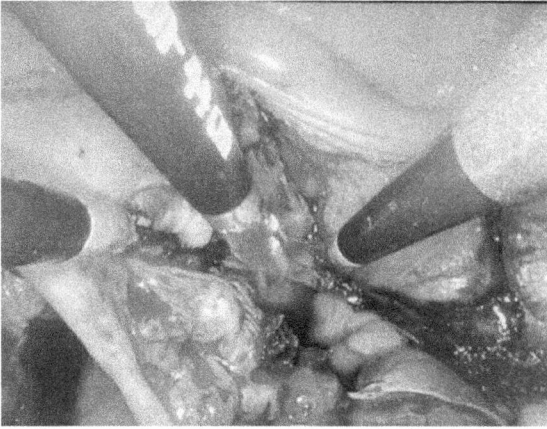

Figure 13.
With the laparoscope in the 30 degree up position, the surgeon's assistant has easy access to the operative field. When the assistant places an instrument, it presents directly between both single site trocars.

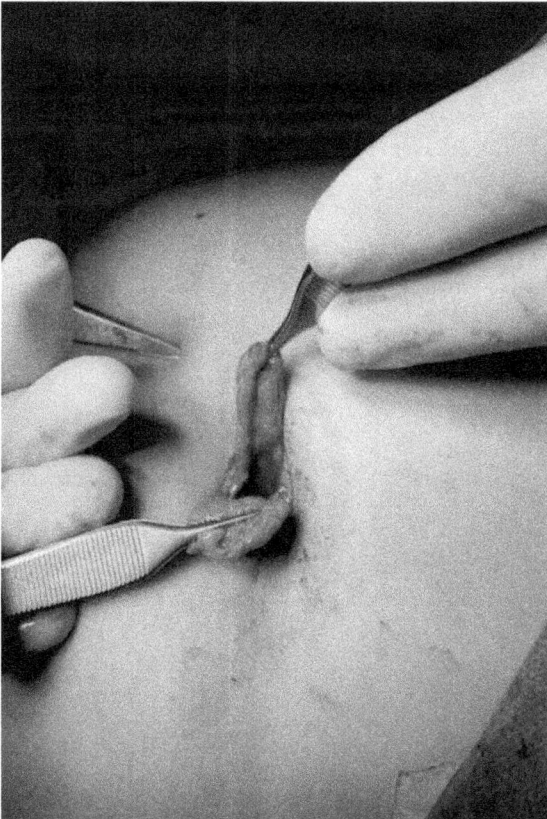

Figure 14.
Skin flaps are created bilaterally by sharply detaching the skin from the fascia until no tension remains.

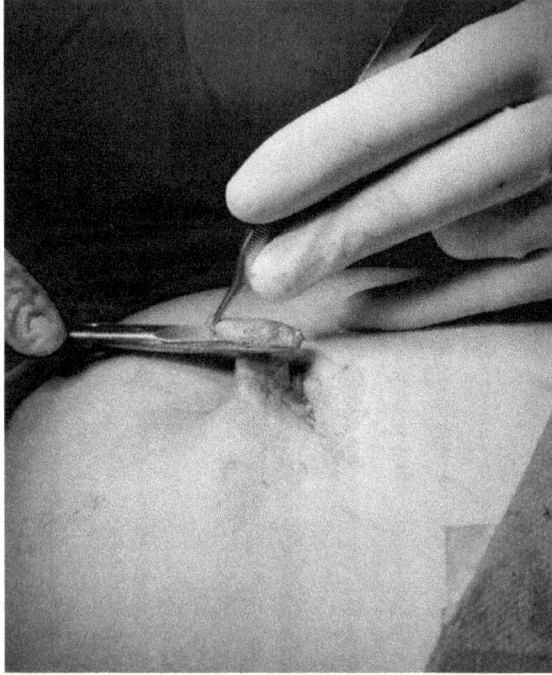

Figure 15.
Redundant skin.

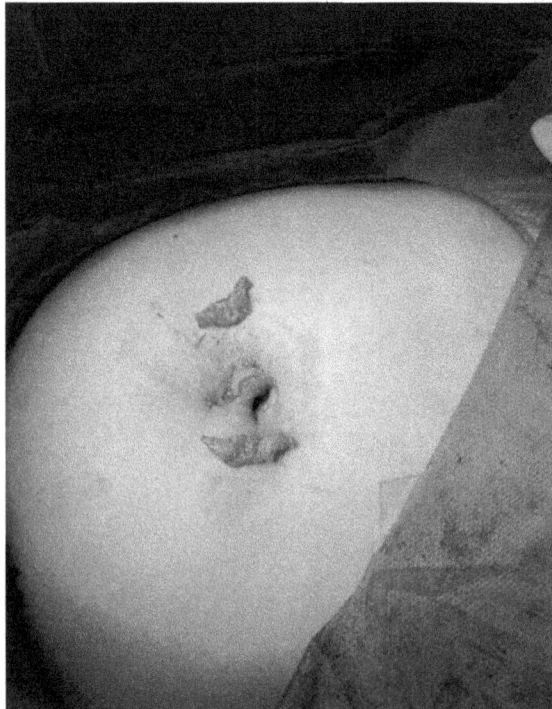

Figure 16.
Redundant skin is trimmed.

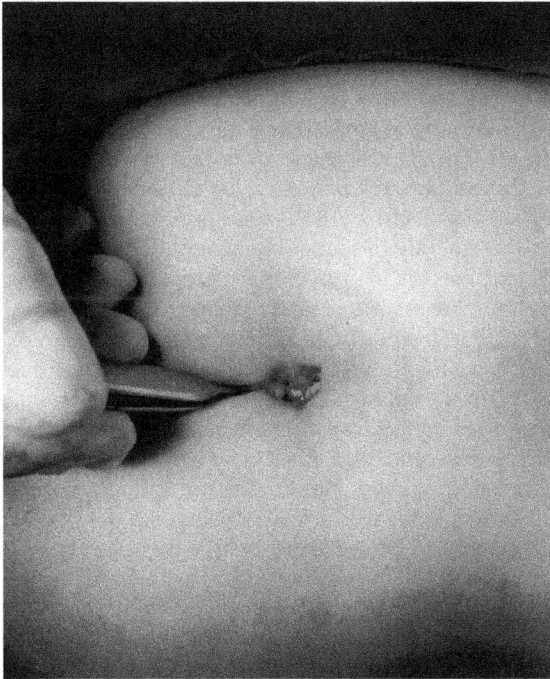

Figure 17.
The skin of both sides of the incision is secured to the fascia with one or two absorbable sutures.

stitch. A deep bite is taken in the fascia to assure that the skin is securely attached. Interrupted inverted 3–0 Vicryl sutures on a cutting needle are then placed in the inferior and superior poles of the incision to reapproximate the skin. Care is taken to include a significant amount of subcutaneous fat with these sutures in order to bulk up the tissue at both poles of the incision (**Figures 13–17**).

A small amount of packing is placed in the umbilicus, and an eye patch trimmed to a 2–3 cm circle is placed over the packing. A medium Tegaderm patch is then placed over the trimmed eye patch. Using a small needle and a 10 ml syringe with reverse suction, the air under the Tegaderm is removed creating a negative pressure dressing. The needle should be placed through the Tegaderm and skin adjacent to the dressing not through the center over the eye patch, otherwise the negative pressure will not be maintained.

10. The utility of the single site robotic system for minor gynecologic surgery

Minor gynecologic surgery generally encompasses surgery on the adnexa and excision of pelvic endometriosis. The single site robotic approach for minor gynecologic surgery offers advantages over both traditional multi-port laparoscopic and robotic surgery. Compared to traditional multi-port surgery, the single site approach is more cosmetic, decreases postoperative pain, and removes the risk of trocar related complications.

In addition, with traditional multi-port laparoscopic or robotic surgery, specimen removal from the abdomen can be challenging. Often one of the incisions needs to be enlarged in order to extract the tissue, resulting in the potential for increased post-operative pain and other wound complications. By contrast, single site robotic surgery provides easy access through the umbilicus for specimen retrieval and morcellation if necessary.

Compared to laparoscopic surgery, both single site and multi-port, the 3D binocular vision and the intuitive ergonomics of the robotic single site platform offer significant advantages. The 3D vision improves dexterity and makes complex ergonomic tasks easier. In addition, the manipulation of tissue is more intuitive with the single site system. This results in more fluid surgical movements and less sword fighting. Finally, although only the single site needle driver is wristed, this compares favorably to laparoscopic instruments that are all uniformly non-wristed.

When contemplating whether to employ the single site robotic approach, consider several factors. First, how difficult is the expected operation. Depending on the surgeon's experience and familiarity with single site surgery, more complex operations may necessitate a multi-port approach. Second, how skilled is the individual surgeon in performing laparoscopic single site surgery. Single site surgery, whether robotic or laparoscopic, virtually always benefits the patient. If a particular surgeon is skilled in laparoscopic single site surgery, this may be a more appropriate technique to use. For an experienced single site surgeon, the laparoscopic approach can be more efficient and can be performed with a slightly smaller umbilical incision.

Ovarian cystectomy is arguably the operation uniquely suited to the robotic single site system. Stripping of an ovarian cyst and suturing the ovary are ergonomically difficult with the laparoscopic single site approach. Multi-port approaches, whether laparoscopic or robotic, may facilitate performing the cystectomy, but they increase the risk for postoperative complications. With the robotic single site approach, the cyst can be easily opened and decompressed. The cyst lining is easily stripped using a grasper and wristed needle driver. Specimen retrieval is easily accomplished through the umbilicus.

For the same reasons, excision of pelvic endometriosis is an operation often well suited to the robotic single site approach. To excise endometriotic implants or explore the pelvic sidewall, significant dexterity is often required. The surgical site is often in a tight space with minimal mobility to the tissue. This creates difficulties even for the experienced laparoscopic single site surgeon.

When first starting to perform robotic single site surgery, the option of adding an additional 8 mm accessory trocar can increase the comfort level of the surgeon. The additional trocar makes all wristed robotic instruments potentially available to assist in the surgery. Eventually, with experience, the extra trocar will become less necessary. Adding the additional trocar mitigates but does not cancel out the benefits of the single site approach. One extra trocar is still better for the patient than 2 or 3 additional ones.

11. Conclusion

The robotic single site system provides a unique surgical approach that can be easily adopted and utilized for gynecologic surgery. It expands the opportunities to perform single surgery beyond just the laparoscopic approach. The single site approach, whether laparoscopic or robotic, virtually always benefits the patient. For the individual surgeon, especially one not particularly comfortable with laparoscopic single site surgery, the robotic single site system can facilitate the transition to single incision surgery as the primary approach to many gynecologic operations. However, even the experienced single site laparoscopic surgeon will find instances where the robotic single site approach is more advantageous.

Author details

John R. Wagner
Board Certified in Obstetrics and Gynecology and Female Pelvic Medicine and
Reconstructive Surgery, New York, USA

*Address all correspondence to: jrwagnermd@yahoo.com

IntechOpen

References

[1] Asakuma M, Komeda K, Yamamoto M, Shimizu T, Iida R, Taniguchi K, Inoue Y, Hirokawa F, Hayashi M, Okuda J, Kondo Y, Uchiyama K. A Concealed "Natural Orifice": Umbilicus Anatomy for Minimally Invasive Surgery. Surg Innov. 2019 Feb;26(1):46-49. doi: 10.1177/1553350618797619. Epub 2018 Sep 7. PMID: 30191768.

[2] C.J. Kliethermes, K. Blazek, B. Nijjar, K. Ali, S.A. Kliethermes, X. Guan, 466 - Pain Outcomes in Single-Incision Laparoscopic Surgery Versus Multiport Hysterectomy, Journal of Minimally Invasive Gynecology, Volume 24, Issue 7, Supplement, 2017, Page S157, ISSN 1553-4650, https://doi.org/10.1016/j.jmig.2017.08.495. (https://www.sciencedirect.com/science/article/pii/S1553465017309366)

[3] Lin Y, Liu M, Ye H, *et al.* Laparoendoscopic single-site surgery compared with conventional laparoscopic surgery for benign ovarian masses: a systematic review and meta-analysis. *BMJ Open* 2020;**10**:e032331. doi: 10.1136/bmjopen-2019-032331.

[4] Song T, Cho J, Kim TJ, Kim IR, Hahm TS, Kim BG, Bae DS. Cosmetic outcomes of laparoendoscopic single-site hysterectomy compared with multi-port surgery: randomized controlled trial. J Minim Invasive Gynecol. 2013 Jul-Aug;20(4):460-7. doi: 10.1016/j.jmig.2013.01.010. Epub 2013 Mar 26. PMID: 23541248.

[5] Hyeong Seok Kim, M.D., et al. Comparison of Single-Incision Robotic Cholecystectomy, Single-Incision Laparoscopic Cholecystectomy and 3-Port Laparoscopic Cholecystectomy - Postoperative Pain, Cosmetic Outcome and Surgeon's Workload. Journal of Minimally Invasive Surgery Vol. 21. No. 4, 2018

[6] Xiaoming Guan, Juan Liu, Yanzhou Wang, Jordan Gisseman, Zhenkun Guan, Christopher Kleithermes, Laparoscopic Single-Incision Supracervical Hysterectomy for an Extremely Large Uterus with Bag Tissue Extraction, Journal of Minimally Invasive Gynecology,Volume 25, Issue 5, 2018,Page 768, ISSN 1553-4650, https://doi.org/10.1016/j.jmig.2017.10.023. (https://www.sciencedirect.com/science/article/pii/S1553465017312591)

Chapter 3

History and Utility of Single Port Laparoscopy, Robotic Assisted Laparoscopy, and Vaginal Laparoscopy (vNOTES) in Gynecologic Surgery

Conor J. Corcoran and Stephen H. Bush

Abstract

Minimally invasive gynecologic surgery is a rapidly growing field, with new modalities and methods being explored constantly. Since the inception of laparoscopic surgery, the goal has been to minimize incision size, which has been further extrapolated to focus on less incisions with Laparoendoscopic Single-site Surgery (LESS). Single site surgery has several advantages, disadvantages, and historically relevant utility. Throughout the ensuing text, the nuances of LESS will be explored and described in detail. Our purpose in this chapter is to explore the history and utility of single site surgery. We hope to set the stage for the extensive coverage and contents of the text to elaborate on LESS and its use in modern Gynecology.

Keywords: minimally invasive surgery, gynecology, surgery, laparoscopy, novel techniques

1. Introduction

From the very beginning, the field of surgery has been full of innovators who have made tireless efforts to optimize and innovate the art form, with each generation of surgeons seeming to reach new heights. The field of minimally invasive gynecologic surgery is no different. These achievements have touched almost all facets of minimally invasive surgery, including laparoscopy, robotic assisted laparoscopy, and natural orifice transluminal endoscopic surgery (NOTES). Laparoscopy has become ubiquitous in gynecologic surgery, most procedures that previously required laparotomy may now be accomplished in this fashion. This is in stark contrast to a few decades ago, where open procedures were the standard of care. Specifically, gynecology in particular has been a forefront for minimally invasive techniques, and one of the quickest specialties to accept laparoscopy. The rapid incorporation of minimally invasive techniques across the specialty of gynecology is likely secondary to two major reasons. First, the relationship between many surgeries and pre-menopausal ovaries leads to a traditionally younger patient population than many other specialties. Second, the exclusively female nature of gynecologic surgery patients means that patients may be more concerned with cosmesis than patients of other specialties.

In that same spirit of advancement, single site surgery has been implemented in Gynecology for the past five decades, with the first single port surgery described as early as 1969 [1]. These "single port" surgeries utilized mono-channel laparoscopic ports with instruments that have sheathed channels built into the polearm. Some physicians still routinely perform this modality of laparoscopy, particularly for tubal occlusion as was originally described in the landmark 1969 case report. The technique was utilized and commonly performed with various tools, ports, and techniques. The culmination, perhaps, was the first single port total laparoscopic hysterectomy, completed in 1991 [2]. For all intents and purposes, procedures similar to this technique dominated single port laparoscopic hysterectomy until 2009 [3, 4], with relatively few other techniques being described.

The modern description of single site laparoscopy revolves around the use of a larger, multichannel port, termed LESS (Laparoendoscopic Single-site Surgery). There were a multitude of studies reported in 2009 with varying methods, results, and outcomes. The general consensus from these texts were that LESS was a feasible and safe surgical method, with no significant increase in perioperative complications. Interestingly, the only field to have documented cases of modern single site surgery prior to gynecology was urology in 2007 [5], which is an intimately related field of medicine.

There are various descriptions of single site techniques. Most authors describe the fundamentals revolving around the concept of an approximately 3 cm umbilical incision into which a larger single port with multiple laparoscopic entry points within that port. Frequently, a wound retractor is placed at this peritoneal entry in order to protect the skin edges and provide an anchor for the port. From here, there are a wide plethora of surgical devices, tools, and specialized equipment described in the literature and surgical textbooks. Importantly, traditional static laparoscopic tools, which are readily available at most surgical theaters, are able to be used as in standard laparoscopy. This allows affordability and ease of access for most surgeons, thus preventing institutional limitations for single site.

LESS procedures have shown promise. Single site has distinct advantages: demonstrating improved cosmesis, decreased blood loss, and decreased complications [6, 7]. While many authors describe different techniques, specimen retrieval is usually facilitated within the single site incision, which may be inherently larger than traditional laparoscopic periumbilical incision. This is incredibly useful in situations where the specimen is large, allowing the surgeon to preoperatively plan a single site procedure if this scenario is anticipated. Those familiar with traditional laparoscopy will know the conundrum of extending the periumbilical incision versus morcellation, which may be circumvented because of the larger fascial incision used in single site procedures.

Of course, there are many drawbacks to single site modalities. These are elucidated in detail throughout this text. The general issues encountered include: instrument clashing, surgeon comfort, inability to triangulate, concerns for hernia rates, and anatomical limitations. Ironically, many of these technical issues were encountered by surgeons with the advent of laparoscopy itself, when open technique was the standard method of operating. Only time and practice will tell if single site surgery will achieve the standardization that other minimally invasive methods have achieved. Thus, most authors feel that we are experiencing a trial period in real clinical applications which will ultimately determine if single port laparoscopy will be a lasting standard or be relegated to the fad of a bygone era by future surgeons.

2. Single site laparoscopy

Interestingly, a large meta-analysis recently showed that across 6 major medical centers, the most common LESS procedure is cholecystectomy [8]. To that end, it has been estimated that 96% of all cholecystectomies are performed laparoscopically [9], which lends itself to being a well-vetted laparoscopic modality ideal for single site surgery. What this overall represents is the rapid progress in all surgical fields in minimally invasive surgery. Indeed, with this growing captivation dominating the surgical fields of medicine, it is ever vital to construct and discuss the various modalities to provide a semblance of standardization. This has historical significance. Look, for example, at the landmark 1929 Richardson hysterectomy paper, which revolutionized hysterectomy technique. It set the tone of a generation of Gynecologists, which alongside antibiotics transformed a surgery that was considered highly dangerous into what is now: a generally safe and routine surgical procedure. It is our responsibility to produce such literature in order advance the field.

While it is evident LESS has mass appeal, the significance of LESS in gynecology is particularly impactful. Its first applications in gynecology can be traced to adnexal surgery after provisional studies demonstrated safety [3, 4]. While its utility is rapidly expanding within the field of gynecology, a contemporary look into the available literature demonstrates a need for ongoing elucidative research.

As discussed above, the term LESS appeared in Gynecologic literature in 2009. LESS has been used for hysterectomy, myomectomy, and gynecologic malignancy. Many modifications have been made since that time and an equally broad assortment of variations have been described. The details of these will be discussed later in this book.

3. Single port robotic

Single port robotic assisted gynecologic surgery was next in the progression of single site procedures in gynecologic surgery. As has been well documented, the LESS procedure is limited by the technical difficulty, loss of triangulation, instrument clashing and reduced visualization. The robotic platform mitigates some of these limitations for single site surgery. The first semi- robotic LESS (R LESS) procedure was reported by Kane and Stepp in 2010 using a SILS port (Covidien, Mansfield, MA) and two ViKY Systems devices (Endocontrol Medical, La Tronche, France) to control the endoscope and vaginal manipulator. A total laparoscopic hysterectomy was then preformed using laparoscopic instruments [10].

The Da Vinci Single Site platform (Intuitive Surgical, Sunnyvale, CA) was approved by the FDA in 2013 for single site gynecologic surgery through the umbilicus. The da Vinci Si Operative system (Intuitive Surgical) compatible platform consists of a 2.5 cm semi-rigid silicone device with five separate lumens. The lumens were originally conceived to include one for the robotic camera, two for the curved robotic instrument sleeves, one for the insufflation port and one for accessory instrumentation administered by an assistant surgeon (**Figure 1**). The curved cannulas allow semi-rigid instruments to be placed through them. This crossing technique effectively reverses the left/right control of the instruments, requiring the device's software to convert the controls for same-sided hand-eye control so the surgeon's contralateral eye is controlling each arm. As a result of this the triangulation issue encountered with non-robotic LESS platforms is much diminished, and there is a notable decrease in instrument clashing.

There are several other single-port devices available for single site access. These include the above mentioned SILS Port Multiple Instrument Access Port (Covidien, Mansfield, MA), as well as GelPort (Applied Medical, Rancho Santa Margarita, CA), and Uni-X Single Port system (Pnavel Systems, Cleveland, OH), and Quad Port (Advanced Surgical Concepts, Bray, Ireland). The GelPort device (**Figure 2**) has been used more recently, for reduced port R-LESS with two incisions. A traditional umbilical incision and one additional lateral abdominal wall incision for one of

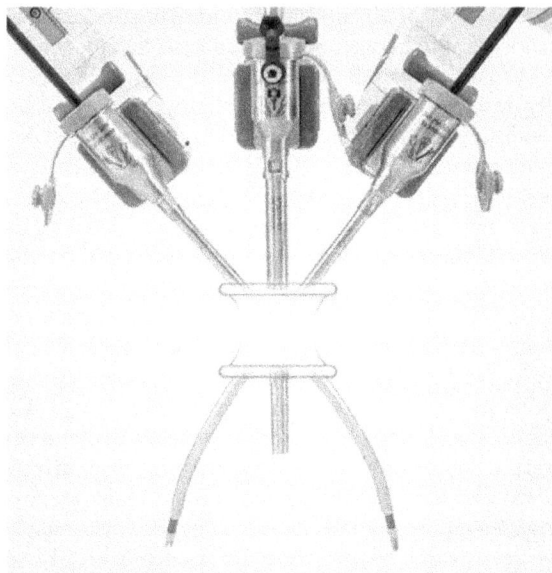

Figure 1.
Depiction of robotic arm positioning and orientation with single site surgery.

the robotic arms, allowing for a robotic laparoscope, instrument and assistant port through the umbilical incision.

The most recent development in R-Less surgery is the approval of the da Vinci SP (Intuitive Surgical, Sunnyvale, CA) platform. This platform was approved by the FDA in the fall of 2018 and was 14 years in development. There is a single 2.5 cm cannula which 3 fully wristed and elbowed instruments as well as a fully wristed endoscope pass. It is able to reach 24 cm in depth and the triangulation occurs at the tip of the instrument. Anatomy can be reached from 360 degrees from one port placement. (**Figure 3**). Although initial data supporting this device for gynecologic surgery is not yet available, there is currently significant utility in urological

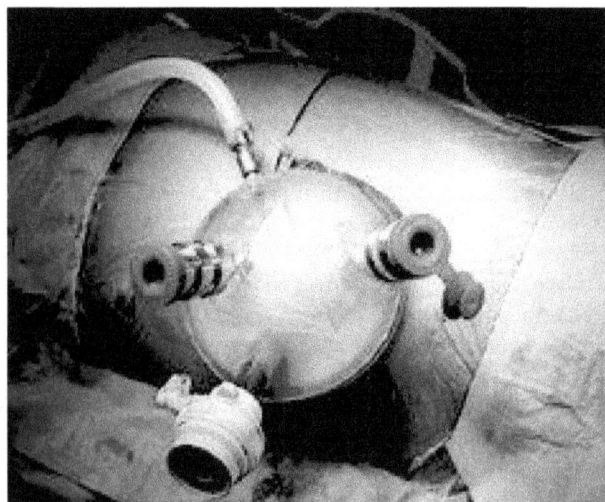

Figure 2.
Single-site Gelport ready for docking.

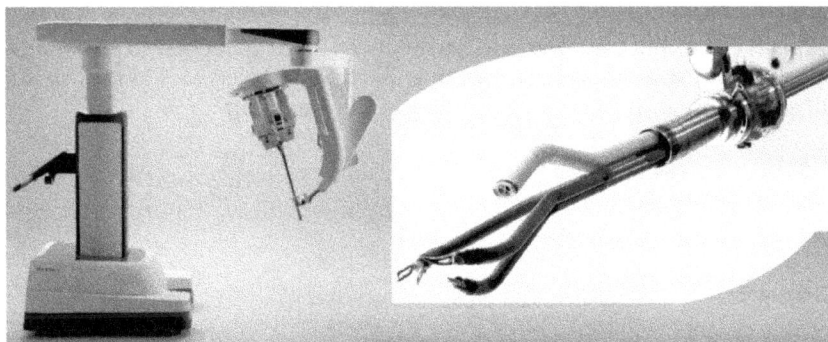

Figure 3.
Single channel robotic arm with multiple instruments.

surgery, and this technology clearly has the potential to further minimize the invasiveness of gynecologic surgery.

4. Vaginal natural orifice transluminal endoscopic surgery (vNOTES)

Natural orifice surgery (NOTES) originated in Gastroenterology/General Surgery circa 2004, utilizing rectal and oral endoscopy to visualize the peritoneum through specific visceral organ sites, such as the fundus of the stomach [11]. NOTES was heralded as a novel method of peritoneal access, subverting the need for skin incisions.

Approximately 10 years later, NOTES has been applied to gynecology by several authors. It was piloted first by Dr. Baekenlandt in the setting of hysterectomy, demonstrating feasibility and safety [12, 13] of the technique. It was developed further for other applications, predominately adnexal surgery via posterior colpotomy while maintaining the uterus. Although there has been limited adoption in the US, this technique has reached faster acceptance internationally, with a high percentage of laparoscopic procedures currently being completed using this method in Taiwan [14–16]. Preliminarily, many early studies have found lower blood loss, shorter hospital stay, and less postoperative pain with vNOTES procedures compared to other accepted modalities [17, 18].

For Gynecologists, it is well known that the vaginal epithelium rapidly heals. Vaginal surgery has been performed safely for generations from vaginal hysterectomies to the historic culdocentesis. In many ways, vaginal surgery has been the conventional "natural orifice" surgery. NOTES, therefore, naturally lent itself to gynecologic surgery. vNOTES is particularly useful for adnexal surgery at the time of vaginal hysterectomy, which offers safe, direct visualization of adjacent anatomy. This is particularly useful in light of the growing evidence suggesting that opportunistic salpingectomy may reduce the risk of epithelial ovarian cancers [17].

While this field is in its infancy in the United States, the technique has great potential to meaningfully impact the field of Gynecology. It combines the techniques of our predecessors with novel technology. In the opinion of some authors, this comes at a critically important time, as the classical vaginal surgical skills in Gynecology are at risk of being lost in many academic settings. Vaginal hysterectomies in general practice and in OB/GYN residencies are decreasing [15, 16] in favor of laparoscopic procedures. This is an unsettling trend, where a procedure that was once the hallmark of gynecologic surgery appears to be phasing out slowly. Many authors suggest that a strong benefit of full acceptance of vNOTES techniques in gynecology will be the maintenance of the vaginal surgery skills. Many consider these skills and techniques of vaginal surgery to be the original first steps towards a minimally invasive culture in gynecology, and that they were seen as the original "calling card" of our field for much of the specialty's existence.

Author details

Conor J. Corcoran[1] and Stephen H. Bush[2*]

1 Charleston Area Medical Center, Charleston, WV, USA

2 Department of Obstetrics and Gynecology, West Virginia University School of Medicine/Charleston Division, Charleston, WV, USA

*Address all correspondence to: shbush@hsc.wvu.edu

IntechOpen

References

[1] Wheeless, CR. "A rapid, inexpensive and effective method of surgical sterilization by laparoscopy". *Journal of reproductive Medicine* 1969. 3;65.

[2] Pelosi, MA. "Laparoscopic hysterectomy with bilateral salpingo-oophrectomy using a single umbilical puncture". *New England Journal of Medicine* 1991. 88(10):721.

[3] Ramirez, P. "Single-port laparoscopic surgery: Is a single incision the next frontier of minimally invasive surgery?". *Gynecologic Oncology* 2009. 114(2):143-144.

[4] Romanelli, J & Earle, D. "Single-port laparoscopic surgery: an overview". *Surg. Endosc*. 2009. 23:1419-1427.

[5] Raman JD, Bensalah K, Bagrodia A, et al. "Laboratory and clinical development of single keyhole umbilical nephrectomy". *Urology* 2007. 70:1039-1042.

[6] Fader, A. & Escobar, P. "Laparoendoscopic single-site surgery (LESS) in gynecologic oncology: technique and initial report". *Gynecol. Oncol*. 2009.

[7] Fagotti, A. *et al*. "Perioperative outcomes of laparoendoscopic single-site surgery (LESS) versus conventional laparoscopy for adnexal disease: a case-control study". *Surg Innov* 2011. 18(1):29-33.

[8] Pfluke, JM *et al*. "Laparoscopic surgery performed through a single incision: a systematic review of the current literature". *Journal of the American College of Surgeons* 212(1):113-118. 2011.

[9] Tsui, C., Klein R, & Garabrant M. "Minimally invasive surgery: national trends in adoption and future directions for hospital strategy." *Surg Endosc*. 2013 Jul;27(7):2253-2257.

[10] Kane, S. & Stepp, KJ. "Laparo-Endoscopic Single-site surgery hysterectomy using lightwight endoscope assistants". *Journal of Robotic Surg*. 2010: 3(4); 253-255.

[11] Kalloo AN, Singh VK, Jagannath SB, et al. "Flexible transgastric peritoneoscopy: a novel approach to diagnostic and therapeutic interventions in the peritoneal cavity". *Gastrointest Endosc* 2004; 60:114.

[12] Baekelandt, J. "Total vaginal NOTES hysterectomy: A New Approach to Hysterectomy". *Journal of Minimally Invasive Gynecology* 2015. 22(6): 1088-1094.

[13] Baekelandt, J *et al*. "Hysterectomy by transvaginal natural orifice transluminal endoscopic surgery versus laparoscopy as a day procedure: a randomized control trial". *BJOG* 2019. 126(1):105-113.

[14] Yang, Y. *et al*. "Transvaginal natural orifice transluminal endoscopic surgery for adnexal masses". *The Journal of Obstetrics and Gynaecology Research* 2013. 39(12); 1604-1609.

[15] Wang, CJ. *et al*. "Learning curve analysis of transvaginal natural orifice transluminal endoscopic hysterectomy". *BMC Surgery*. 2019. 19(88).

[16] H. Su, *et al*. "Hysterectomy via transvaginal natural orifice transluminal endoscopic surgery (NOTES): feasibility of an innovative approach". *Taiwan J Obstet Gynecol* 2012. 51; 217-221.

[17] Wright, J et al. "Nationwide trands in the performance of inpatient hysterectomy in the United States". *Obstetrical Gynecology* 2013;122:233-241.

[18] ACOG Committee Opinion 744. "Opportunistic Salpingectomy as a Strategy for Epithelial Cancer prevention." *Obstet Gynecol* 2019; 133 e279-e284.

Chapter 4

Single Port Laparoscopic Assisted Hysterectomy

Michael L. Nimaroff and Eric Crihfield

Abstract

This chapter describes the necessary steps to perform single port laparoscopic hysterectomy. This surgical approach is an innovative method to offer all of the benefits of multi-port laparoscopy through one single incision usually in and around the umbilicus. Using core surgical principles and instruments available for single port surgery external triangulation and full range of motion can be maintained to achieve the required internal manipulation of instruments and tissue dissection. All single port surgeries require a specialized port used along with an angled or flexible laparoscope for visualization. Traditional laparoscopic instruments may be used for the surgical dissection and completion of the procedure.

Keywords: single port, laparoscopic surgery, LESS, single site surgery

1. Introduction

Laparoscopic hysterectomy was first described in 1989 and, with its superior surgical results and outcome metrics compared to the abdominal route, the number of laparoscopic hysterectomies has increased significantly over the past three decades [1–3]. Additionally, investments in product development over the last thirty years has further supported adoption of the procedure and the birth of the field of minimally invasive surgery in general. In gynecology, acceptance of the technique in all surgical subspecialties has further helped drive the increased procedure volume even when dealing with complex pathology. The improvements in surgical outcomes over the abdominal route demonstrated with all forms of laparoscopic surgery or, any minimally invasive approach, has led to further innovation in the minimally invasive field and the birth of single port access surgery (SPA). Single port surgery was developed in an effort to further decrease the invasiveness of the procedure and maximize the benefits of laparoscopy [4, 5].

Single port access surgery, as its name implies, is a route of laparoscopic surgery that involves performing the entire procedure through one incision and one port (as opposed to the usual 3–5), usually at the umbilicus, that is generally 2–3 cm in length [6]. This route of surgery goes by many names including SPA, laparoendoscopic single-site surgery (LESS), single-site laparoscopic (SSL), single-port laparoscopy (SPLS), and single incision laparoscopic surgery (SILS) amongst others, with SILS and LESS the two most common nomenclatures used [7]. However, all of the above names are acceptable and indicate the identical surgical procedure. The first single port laparoscopic hysterectomy was described in 1991, but did not gain initial acceptance likely due to both the steep learning curve required and the lack of appropriate instrumentation available at the time. The route did not begin to gain popularity until general surgery began publishing about SILS cholecystectomies and appendectomies in the mid-2000s [4, 5]. The main advantage to single port hysterectomy over the traditional laparoscopic approach is cosmetic, as the incision needed can often be well hidden in the umbilicus [6, 8]. There is also evidence that this route may reduce pain and result in a faster recovery for the patient [6, 8]. These improved outcomes must be balanced with the potential disadvantages of single port compared to multi-port laparoscopy, resulting from the technical challenges of the procedure. Having all the instruments passing through the same port site can certainly make the procedure more challenging due to instrument crowding, limits on visualization, and loss of triangulation [6, 8]. There is also some concern that the larger incision required may be more at risk for wound complications and hernias [6, 8]. However, with appropriate instrumentation and surgical technique these limitations can managed and overcome. Here we will review the key principles, strategies, and available instrumentation that can help mitigate the challenges of single port hysterectomy, as well as, discuss the clinical outcomes data comparing single port hysterectomy to multi-port hysterectomy.

2. Patient selection

Performing any new surgical technique requires education, observation, and/or simulation/proctoring before attempting the surgical approach independently. In addition, appropriate patient selection is key to achieving early success. Single port hysterectomy certainly falls into this category and once completing your education and training process, the surgeon should initially perform SPA adnexal surgery successfully before attempting hysterectomy. Also, patient selection is critical in achieving early success with this approach. During the surgeons first 5–10 cases limiting procedures to patients without a history of pelvic (especially cesarean sections) or gastrointestinal tract surgery and with less complex pelvic pathology (ie. fibroids < 14 weeks size, no history of endometriosis). However, after gaining experience with the technique, the proficient surgeon can use this approach with virtually the same patients and pathology as can be addressed with multi-port laparoscopy. Even with experience the single port dissection of an adherent bladder and approaching a very large and distorted fibroid uterus can be challenging and one should never hesitate to add an additional 5 mm port if necessary.

3. Procedure

The surgical approach to single port hysterectomy is based on two fundamental principles: 1. The need for external triangulation of the surgical instruments to avoid internal clashing and 2. Viewing the internal procedure (video monitor) should appear identical to the view seen with any other multi-port laparoscopic procedure. These two principles are the key foundation to performing safe and successful SPA hysterectomies. Accomplishing the above principles begins with port selection. Over the past decade we have seen a number of ports developed for this procedure, however, we currently prefer the GelPOINT Mini (Applied Medical Corporation) and use this port with virtually all types of single port surgeries (**Figure 1**).

This port provides tremendous flexibility for instrument insertion, ability to triangulate, and ease of specimen removal when performing laparoscopic supracervical hysterectomy (**Figure 2**).

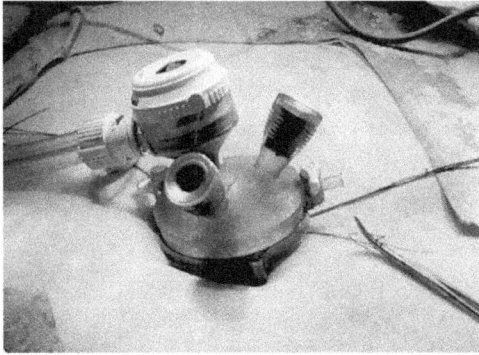

Figure 1.
GelPOINT mini in the umbilicus.

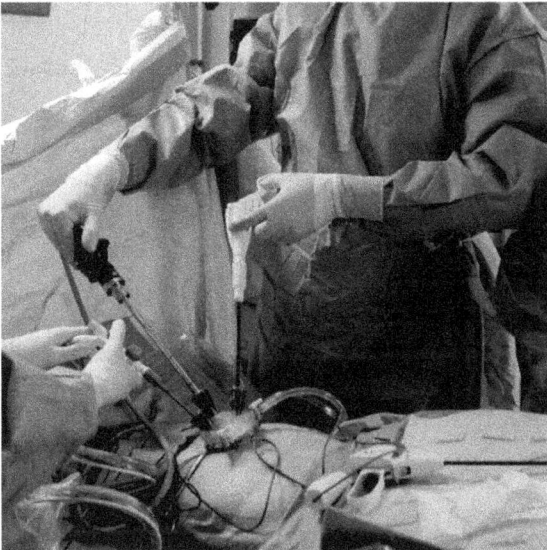

Figure 2.
External triangulation creates the necessary spacing to prevent clashing of instruments both inside and outside of the body.

Performing single port hysterectomy requires the patient to be placed in dorsal lithotomy with placement of a uterine manipulator if possible. When approaching a large myomatous uterus the manipulation and traction may be accomplished from above using either a myoma screw or laparoscopic tenaculum, however, when possible manipulating from below is preferable. The patient should have both arms tucked at the side and secured per routine for placement in trendelenburg positioning. The SPA port can be placed anywhere in the upper abdomen but typically is placed in the umbilicus for superior cosmetic results. The skin incision may be periumbilical, directly in the midline of the umbilicus, or inserted through an omega incision just inside the lower ridge of the umbilicus (**Figure 3**). With an omega incision a 2 cm fascial incision is made transversely below the skin incision and the fascia is tagged with two interrupted sutures at both angles to aid both in port insertion and closure when the procedure is completed (**Figures 4** and **5**). An omega incision is preferable for superior cosmetic result and the ability to close a

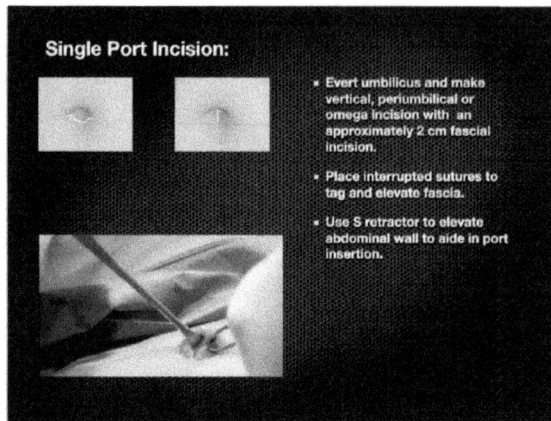

Figure 3.
Single port incision options.

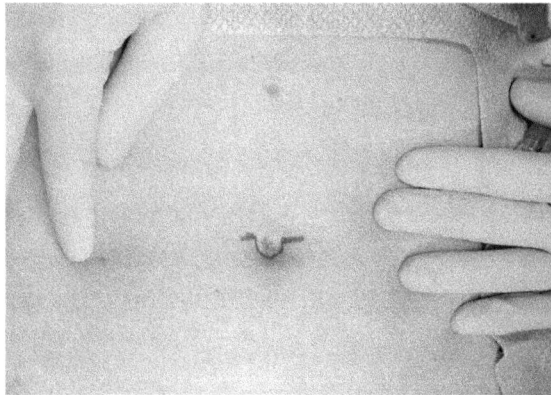

Figure 4.
Outline of omega incision.

well-developed transverse fascial layer that is found subumbilical and below the skin incision, in contrast to the less prominent fascial layer found when going directly through the midline of the umbilicus.

The port is inserted after the peritoneal cavity is entered and digital and visual inspection is satisfied for the absence of abdominal wall adhesions. See **Table 1** for the list of recommended instrumentation needed for the successful completion of a single port hysterectomy. A zero degree laparoscope should not be considered and the surgeon must use a 30 degree, 45 degree, or flexible scope to obtain the necessary external triangulation and internal visualization to complete the procedure easily (**Figure 6**).

The accessory instruments may be rigid or one may use flexible graspers, scissors, and vessel sealers if available at your institution, however, the procedure can be accomplished without additional flexible or angled instruments except for angled or flexible laparoscope. The hysterectomy is performed using the same surgical technique as is used with any multi-port approach including a retroperitoneal dissection and ureteral identification as indicated. To review, the basic setup and instruments needed for single port hysterectomy begins with the patient in dorsal lithotomy with both arms tucked at the side. Next an angled or flexible low

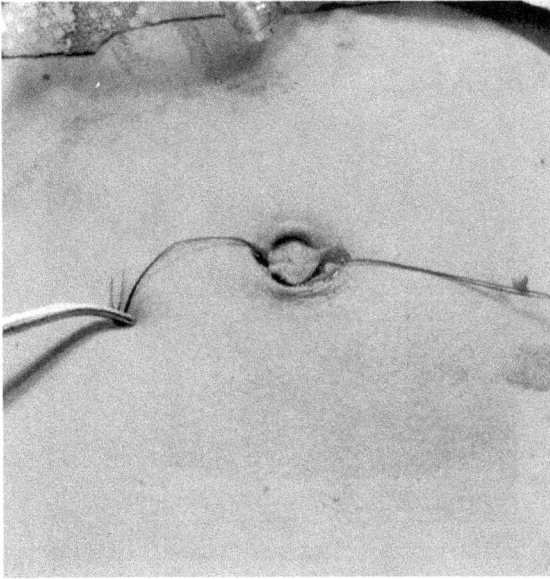

Figure 5.
Omega incision with two sutures tagging the fascia.

>*SPA port*
>*30,45 degree or flexible laparoscope*
>*uterine manipulator*
>*vessel sealer*
>*articulating grasper (if available)*
>*bipolar forceps*

Table 1.
Single port hysterectomy instrumentation.

profile scope (the light cord cannot attach at 90 degrees) must be used in addition to the selected single port. The remaining accessory instruments may be traditional devices preferred by the individual surgeon. In order to achieve adequate spacing for external triangulation and creating the necessary room for both external and internal range of motion, the camera should always be positioned in the midline port and instruments used for dissection and coagulation should be placed and approached from the contralateral side (**Figure 2**). In keeping with these key principles when performing single port procedures and, especially, hysterectomy when deviating the specimen laterally to the right the vessel sealer is inserted on the contralateral side (right to secure the left sided pelvic vessels) and the grasper (or tenaculum) is placed on the ipsilateral side. This approach ensures sufficient external triangulation (**Figure 7**).

The remainder of the dissection is approached using these same principles. Following dissection of the bladder peritoneum and securing the uterine vessels the colpotomy is made using a hook cautery, bipolar spatula, or harmonics (**Figures 8** and **9**).

Following removal of the specimen the colpotomy can be closed either transvaginally or from above, an extremely difficult challenge for even the most experienced surgeon. Alternatively, the surgeon can use a 2 mm needle grasper placed anywhere desired in the lower abdomen to aid in colpotomy closure from above (**Figure 10**).

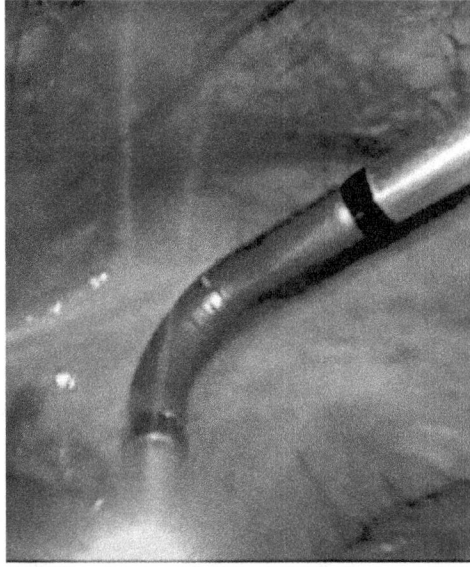

Figure 6.
Flexible laparoscope provides 360 degrees of visualization.

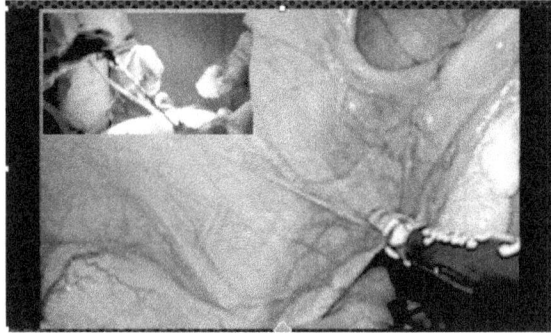

Figure 7.
The left infundibulopelvic ligament is secured by placing the vessel sealer through the contralateral port (right).

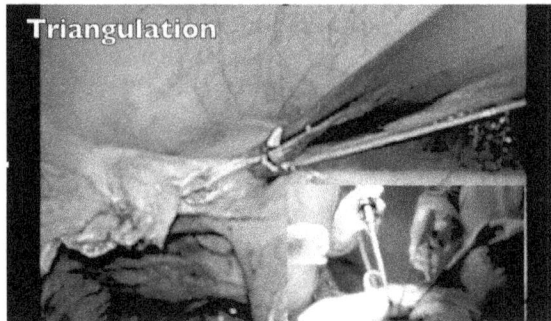

Figure 8.
Triangulation is achieved by placing the grasper on the left to deviate the uterus to the right. The left anterior bladder peritoneum is approached from the right port.

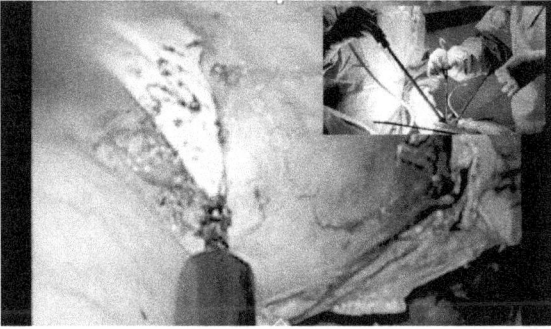

Figure 9.
Colpotomy incision.

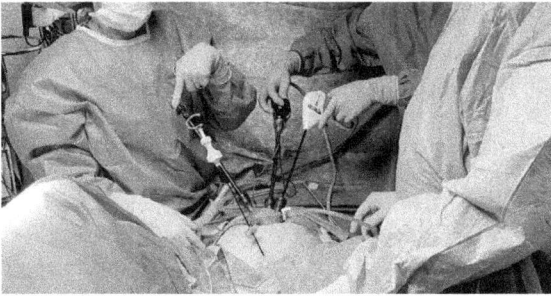

Figure 10.
Needle grasper placed suprapubically to assist with SPA hysterectomy.

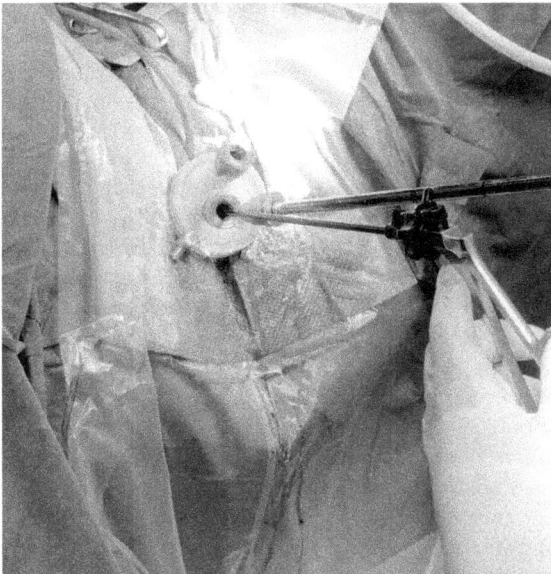

Figure 11.
VNOTES (vaginal natural orifice trans-luminal endoscopic surgery) hysterectomy.

Approaching the colpotomy closure form above standard laparoscopic instruments can be used, however, using both a self righting needle driver and an articulating grasper aids in colpotomy closure but these tools are not mandatory.

Prior to completing the procedure lower the abdominal pressure to inspect for bleeding before removing the port and closing the fascia. Once mastering single port hysterectomy from above a similar approach can be used to perform the procedure transvaginally using similar instrumentation (**Figure 11**). This procedure is called total hysterectomy by transvaginal natural orifice trans-luminal endoscopic surgical approach (VNOTES). The procedure begins as a traditional vaginal hysterectomy but following the creation of the anterior and posterior colpotomies and securing the uterosacral ligaments the single port is inserted and the remainder of the procedure performed via the laparoscope from below [9, 10]. With advancing experience and comfort virtually all forms of hysterectomy can be approached using the single port approach including radical hysterectomy [11, 12].

4. Discussion

When discussing SPA hysterectomies it is important to note that across surgical fields the safety of single port access surgery is well documented with most studies demonstrating equivalent rates of complications when compared to standard laparoscopy [8]. Aside from improved cosmesis, the benefits over multi-port laparoscopy are less well documented, and there is concern that the benefits may not be worth the increase in technical difficulty. In most cases these challenges can be overcome using the appropriate technique, instrumentation, and experience the outcomes of single port hysterectomy can match those achieved with multi-port hysterectomy. Additionally, it is critical to adhere to the core principles outlined above. In a study that evaluated the learning curve for SPA in TLH-BSO found that a significant improvement in operative time was attained after 10 cases (from 79.4 minutes to 56.8 minutes), with modest improvements after 20 cases [13]. A retrospective study of 190 laparoscopic supracervical hysterectomies with manual morcellation found that for uteri with a median weight of 245 g (range 100-1960 g), the median total operative time was 69 minutes (range 36–183 minutes) [14]. One RCT and a few observational studies that have looked at operative time for single port hysterectomy have found no significant difference in operative time when compared to multi-port hysterectomy [4, 5, 15]. A recent retrospective study looking at robotic single port surgery compared to conventional single port found an average decrease in operative time of 18 minutes that was statistically significant [16]. Expert single port surgeons have also demonstrated the feasibility of removing uteri as big as 20 weeks size when using articulating instruments [17]. One systematic review did however show an increased rate of "procedure failure" with single port hysterectomy, with an odds ratio of conversion to different route of 3.95 for single port hysterectomy [3]. However, of the 58 conversions amongst 1617 single port hysterectomies evaluated, 40 of them were conversion to multi-port laparoscopy with only 18 being conversion to open, compared to 7 of 1923 multi-port laparoscopic hysterectomies being converted to open. Conversion rate to open procedure was not statistically evaluated in their analysis. Overall, the literature generally demonstrates that single port hysterectomy can be accomplished efficiently with an appropriately experienced surgeon.

Several case reports and pilot studies have additionally demonstrated the feasibility in using single port for hysterectomy and lymph node dissection in low risk/ early stage endometrial cancer both with the DaVinci robotic single port platform and with conventional single port [18–22]. The largest study available on single port in gynecologic oncology cases out of the Cleveland Clinic was a retrospective study that, amongst cases for other pathology, included 339 cases for endometrial hyperplasia or malignancy [23]. Of patients included, 126 underwent a pelvic lymphadenectomy and 67 patients had a para-aortic lymphadenectomy. Their outcomes had a low rate of conversion at 3.2% with the addition of a hand-assist port in 5.0% of patients (22% of those were planned from the start of the case), though the study did not specify how many of those conversions were in the 339 endometrial pathology cases as the total n of the study was 908. The authors concluded that single port access surgery was safe and feasible in gynecologic malignant and premalignant conditions with a low rate of adverse outcomes. The most prevalent complication was incisional hernias at a rate of 5.5%, with higher rates being seen in patients with comorbidities such as obesity and diabetes. These studies show promising results in regards to surgical techniques and complication rates, but at this time there is limited evidence that evaluates the long term outcomes of disease free survival in endometrial cancer patients undergoing single port surgery when compared to multi-port laparoscopy.

Looking further into improved patient outcomes with single port access surgery, studies have shown some improvement in pain and satisfaction, but others report mixed results. In one RCT (n = 100) and another prospective cohort study (n = 70) both showed a significant decrease in pain levels for single port hysterectomy [4, 5]. However, a meta-analysis of RCTs for any laparoscopic gynecologic procedure and a meta-analysis of adnexal surgery found no difference in pain between single port access surgery and multi-port laparoscopy [24, 25]. Regarding patient satisfaction, a small RCT (n = 108) that looked at multiple outcomes for single port hysterectomy compared to four-port hysterectomy found increased patient satisfaction (93.8% vs. 89.5%), as well as decreased infection rate (1/52 vs. 5/56) and shorter duration of immobilization (14.6 hours vs. 15.7 hours) for single port hysterectomy compared to four-port [26]. One of the most consistent positive results for single port surgery is improved cosmetic results. Multiple studies have found improved cosmetics scores after single-incision hysterectomy when compared to multi-port both in the short and long term [27–29]. One of the biggest concerns with single port is incisional hernias, and while some smaller studies have not been able to find a difference, the most recent large meta-analysis that included both gynecologic and general surgery procedures did find an increased rate of incisional hernias with single port surgery (odds ratio 2.83), however the overall rate of the complication was low (1.69% for SILS vs. 0.39% for multi-port) and there was no statistically significant difference in the rate of hernias that requires surgical repair [30]. Also, key to avoiding postoperative incisional hernia is performing the initial incision and port insertion in an area with adequate fascia for closure. This is one potential limitation for direct midline umbilical insertions.

Given the comparable safety and outcomes, when considering performing a hysterectomy via single incision, the decision to use this approach will ultimately depend on both surgeon experience and patient medical history and pathology. With enough experience, single port hysterectomy is feasible and efficient making it comparable to multi-port for the right candidate. In terms of outcomes, cosmetic results are most consistently improved, while other outcomes are comparable to multi-port laparoscopic hysterectomy. These outcomes should be taken in consideration and discussed with the patient, and a shared-decision making process can help individualize the best route of surgery for each case.

Author details

Michael L. Nimaroff[1,2]* and Eric Crihfield[2]

1 Department of Obstetrics and Gynecology, Donald and Barbara Zucker School of Medicine at Hofstra/Northwell, Hempstead, NY, USA

2 Department of Obstetrics and Gynecology North Shore University Hospital and Long Island Jewish Medical Center

*Address all correspondence to: mnimaroff@northwell.edu

IntechOpen

References

[1] Dedden SJ, Geomini PMAJ, Huirne JAF, Bongers MY. Vaginal and Laparoscopic hysterectomy as an outpatient procedure: A systematic review. *Eur J Obstet Gynecol Reprod Biol*. 2017;216:212-223. doi:10.1016/j.ejogrb.2017.07.015

[2] Atkin RP, Nimaroff ML, Bhavsar V. Applying single-incision laparoscopic surgery to gyn practice: What's involved. *OBG Manag*. 2011;23(4):28-36.

[3] Yang L, Gao J, Zeng L, Weng Z, Luo S. Systematic review and meta-analysis of single-port versus conventional laparoscopic hysterectomy. *Int J Gynaecol Obstet*. 2016;133(1):9-16. doi:10.1016/j.ijgo.2015.08.013

[4] Chen Y-J, Wang P-H, Ocampo EJ, Twu N-F, Yen M-S, Chao K-C. Single-port compared with conventional laparoscopic-assisted vaginal hysterectomy: a randomized controlled trial. *Obstet Gynecol*. 2011;117(4):906-912. doi:10.1097/AOG.0b013e31820c666a

[5] Kliethermes C, Blazek K, Ali K, Nijjar JB, Kliethermes S, Guan X. Postoperative Pain After Single-Site Versus Multiport Hysterectomy. *JSLS*. 2017;21(4). doi:10.4293/JSLS.2017.00065

[6] Hoffman BL, Schorge JO, Halvorson LM, Hamid CA, Corton MM, Schaffer JI. Minimally Invasive Surgery Fundamentals. In: *Williams Gynecology, 4e*. McGraw-Hill Education; 2020. Accessed August 24, 2020. accessmedicine.mhmedical.com/content.aspx?aid=1171665604

[7] Pryor A, Bates AT. Abdominal access techniques used in laparoscopic surgery. In: Post TedW, ed. *UpToDate*. UpToDate; 2020. https://www.uptodate.com/contents/abdominal-access-techniques-used-in-laparoscopic-surgery

[8] Spight DH, Jobe BA, Hunter JG. Minimally Invasive Surgery, Robotics, Natural Orifice Transluminal Endoscopic Surgery, and Single-Incision Laparoscopic Surgery. In: Brunicardi FC, Andersen DK, Billiar TR, et al., eds. *Schwartz's Principles of Surgery, 11e*. McGraw-Hill Education; 2019. Accessed August 24, 2020. accessmedicine.mhmedical.com/content.aspx?aid=1164309103

[9] Nulens K, Bosteels J, De Rop C, Baekelandt J. vNOTES Hysterectomy for Large Uteri: A Retrospective Cohort Study of 114 Patients. *J Minim Invasive Gynecol*. Published online October 14, 2020. doi:10.1016/j.jmig.2020.10.003

[10] Housmans S, Noori N, Kapurubandara S, et al. Systematic Review and Meta-Analysis on Hysterectomy by Vaginal Natural Orifice Transluminal Endoscopic Surgery (vNOTES) Compared to Laparoscopic Hysterectomy for Benign Indications. *J Clin Med*. 2020;9(12). doi:10.3390/jcm9123959

[11] Boruta DM, Fagotti A, Bradford LS, et al. Laparoendoscopic single-site radical hysterectomy with pelvic lymphadenectomy: initial multi-institutional experience for treatment of invasive cervical cancer. *J Minim Invasive Gynecol*. 2014;21(3):394-398. doi:10.1016/j.jmig.2013.10.005

[12] Chen S, Qi X, Chen L, et al. Laparoendoscopic Single-site Radical Hysterectomy: Sufficient Exposure via Effective Suspension. *J Minim Invasive Gynecol*. 2020;27(4):809-810. doi:10.1016/j.jmig.2019.08.030

[13] Fader AN, Cohen S, Escobar PF, Gunderson C. Laparoendoscopic single-site surgery in gynecology. *Curr Opin Obstet Gynecol*. 2010;22(4):331-338. doi:10.1097/GCO.0b013e32833be979

[14] Chang Y, Kay N, Huang MR, Huang SJ, Tsai EM. Laparoendoscopic Single-Site Supracervical Hysterectomy with Manual Morcellation: A Retrospective Study. *J Minim Invasive Gynecol*. 2018;25(6):1094-1100. doi:10.1016/j.jmig.2018.02.017

[15] Murji A, Patel VI, Leyland N, Choi M. Single-incision laparoscopy in gynecologic surgery: a systematic review and meta-analysis. *Obstet Gynecol*. 2013;121(4):819-828. doi:10.1097/AOG.0b013e318288828c

[16] Zhang Y, Kohn JR, Guan X. Single-Incision Hysterectomy Outcomes With and Without Robotic Assistance. *JSLS*. 2019;23(4). doi:10.4293/JSLS.2019.00046

[17] Guan X, Liu J, Wang Y, Gisseman J, Guan Z, Kleithermes C. *Laparoscopic Single-Incision Supracervical Hysterectomy for an Extremely Large Uterus with Bag Tissue Extraction*. Vol 25.; 2018. doi:10.1016/j.jmig.2017.10.023

[18] Vizza E, Corrado G, Mancini E, et al. Robotic single-site hysterectomy in low risk endometrial cancer: a pilot study. *Ann Surg Oncol*. 2013;20(8):2759-2764. doi:10.1245/s10434-013-2922-9

[19] Yoon A, Yoo H-N, Lee Y-Y, et al. *Robotic Single-Port Hysterectomy, Adnexectomy, and Lymphadenectomy in Endometrial Cancer*. Vol 22.; 2015. doi:10.1016/j.jmig.2014.12.003

[20] Sinno AK, Fader AN, Tanner EJ 3rd. *Single Site Robotic Sentinel Lymph Node Biopsy and Hysterectomy in Endometrial Cancer*. Vol 137.; 2015. doi:10.1016/j.ygyno.2014.12.033

[21] Fanfani F, Rossitto C, Gagliardi ML, et al. Total laparoendoscopic single-site surgery (LESS) hysterectomy in low-risk early endometrial cancer: a pilot study. *Surg Endosc*. 2012;26(1):41-46. doi:10.1007/s00464-011-1825-8

[22] Demirayak G, Comba C, Özdemir İA. *Laparoendoscopic Single-Site Sentinel Lymph Node Detection in Endometrial Cancer*. Vol 25.; 2018. doi:10.1016/j.jmig.2017.10.035

[23] Moulton L, Jernigan AM, Carr C, Freeman L, Escobar PF, Michener CM. Single-port laparoscopy in gynecologic oncology: seven years of experience at a single institution. *Am J Obstet Gynecol*. 2017;217(5):610.e1-610.e8. doi:10.1016/j.ajog.2017.06.008

[24] Schmitt A, Crochet P, Knight S, Tourette C, Loundou A, Agostini A. Single-Port Laparoscopy vs Conventional Laparoscopy in Benign Adnexal Diseases: A Systematic Review and Meta-Analysis. *J Minim Invasive Gynecol*. 2017;24(7):1083-1095. doi:10.1016/j.jmig.2017.07.001

[25] Pontis A, Sedda F, Mereu L, et al. Review and meta-analysis of prospective randomized controlled trials (RCTs) comparing laparo-endoscopic single site and multiport laparoscopy in gynecologic operative procedures. *Arch Gynecol Obstet*. 2016;294(3):567-577. doi:10.1007/s00404-016-4108-8

[26] Li M, Han Y, Feng YC. Single-port laparoscopic hysterectomy versus conventional laparoscopic hysterectomy: a prospective randomized trial. *J Int Med Res*. 2012;40(2):701-708. doi:10.1177/147323001204000234

[27] Demirayak G, Özdemir İA, Comba C, et al. Comparison of laparoendoscopic single-site (LESS) surgery and conventional multiport laparoscopic (CMPL) surgery for hysterectomy: long-term outcomes of abdominal incisional scar. *J Obstet Gynaecol*. 2020;40(2):217-221. doi:10.1080/01443615.2019.1606183

[28] Song T, Cho J, Kim T-J, et al. Cosmetic outcomes of laparoendoscopic

single-site hysterectomy compared
with multi-port surgery: randomized
controlled trial. *J Minim Invasive
Gynecol*. 2013;20(4):460-467.
doi:10.1016/j.jmig.2013.01.010

[29] Yeung PPJ, Bolden CR, Westreich D,
Sobolewski C. Patient preferences of
cosmesis for abdominal incisions in
gynecologic surgery. *J Minim Invasive
Gynecol*. 2013;20(1):79-84. doi:10.1016/j.
jmig.2012.09.008

[30] Connell MB, Selvam R, Patel SV.
Incidence of incisional hernias following
single-incision versus traditional
laparoscopic surgery: a meta-analysis.
Hernia. 2019;23(1):91-100. doi:10.1007/
s10029-018-1853-6

Chapter 5

Robotic Laparoscopic Single-Site Surgery

Rene I. Luna

Abstract

Minimally invasive surgery has changed the landscape of women's surgical healthcare. Conventional and robotic laparoscopy are the preferred approach for many major minimally invasive gynecological procedures. However, the philosophy of minimally invasive surgery has been pushed to reduce the size and minimize the number of ports placed. Many conventional minimally invasive surgical procedures use 3–5 ports through multiple small incisions. Laparoscopic single site surgery tries to perform on that philosophy but has its limitations. Enters robotic surgery already a major force in minimally invasive surgery and now sets to remove the limitations of single site surgery. However it requires proper understanding of the instruments and the techniques for successful robotic single site surgery. It starts with patient selection. Knowing the instruments needed and the proper set up of those instruments. Then knowing how to use the instruments in operating and suturing and closing. And finish with special considerations.

Keywords: robotic single-site, patient selection, set up, port entry, instruments, first assist and closure, special considerations

1. Introduction

Minimally invasive surgery has changed the landscape of women's surgical healthcare. Women are now able to undergo major surgeries as outpatient procedures leading to faster recoveries and more importantly, faster return to normalcy. Conventional and robotic laparoscopy are now the preferred approach for many major minimally invasive gynecological procedures. The predictable result has been a change in the overall philosophy of minimally invasive surgery in gynecology today. This philosophy constantly pushes to reduce the size of each trocar port and to minimize the number of ports placed. Currently, many conventional minimally invasive surgical procedures use 3–5 ports through multiple small incisions. Each port carries a small, but not statistically zero risk for a port site complication [1]. These port site complications may include bleeding, infection, organ injury, soft tissue trauma (leading to increased post op pain,) the risk of herniation and decreased final cosmesis [2].

Now with new instrumentation, as well as better visualization and greater surgeon dedication, procedures can be performed using a single incision port entry. This leads to often entirely concealing the incision at the umbilicus. The result is rewarding the patient and surgeon with a virtually scarless procedure [3].

This is not to say, however, that no challenges remain. Some of these new challenges Include mastering inline camera viewing, off center operating, the difficulty

Instruments Needed for Robotic Single Port Hysterectomy
30-degree robotic scope in downward position
Intuitive Gelport™
Intuitive right and left curved trocars
Fenestrated Bipolar grasper
Monopolar hook
Single site wristed needle driver
AirSeal™ insufflator
8 mm AirSeal™ port
Bariatric suction tip
Barbed 2.0 trimethylene carbonate suture on a P14 reverse cutting needle V-Loc™
Uterine manipulator (surgeon's preference on type used)

Table 1.
Instruments needed for robotic single port hysterectomy.

of instrument crowding and a lack of instrument triangulation resulting in techni-cally challenging laparoscopic single-site surgery. To try and improve on these challenges, the only commercially available system currently available, The Intuitive Robotic Surgical System™ comes equipped with a single-site robotic instrument set on their Si and Xi models. The Robotic single-site instruments provide and enable a broader range of instrument movement with flexible instruments which allows them to fit into curved trocars. The result is greatly improved triangulation and almost a complete elimination of instrument crowding. These changes significantly improve surgical movements allowing the surgeon to have greater motion and technical ease of operating. The surgeon has complete control of the camera and instruments and remains sitting at a comfortable surgeon console. This provides an extremely ergonomically friendly procedure, almost regardless of surgical time [4, 5]. This procedure, however, is not without its own challenges.

In the following sections, we will discuss patient evaluation, instruments needed, and some important differences between robotic multiport and robot single-site surgery. Further along we will go through the sequence of steps neces-sary for port placement and docking while performing a robotic single-site hyster-ectomy. We will then finish by discussing special considerations (**Table 1**).

2. Patient evaluation

The process of deciding the appropriate surgical route remains as recom-mended by the American College of Obstetricians and Gynecologists [6]. This generally means that a diligent surgeon should take into account the individual circumstances of the patient, along with the patient's medical and surgical histo-ries, as include consideration of the particular surgeon's own skills as well as the modalities available prior to deciding on the final surgical route. However, when beginning robotic single-site surgery, patient selection is an even more important process. Patients with a body mass index (BMI) of less than 32 to 34 are going to be the best candidates due to the height of the single-site port trocar and the complex nature of laparoscopic surgery in more obese patients. An initial uterine size of 12 cm or smaller in length will also be ideal for port placement and maximize the comfortable range of instrument movements. A larger uterus will significantly limit both of these aspects, requiring more advanced maneuvers to proceed. Also, a patient's surgical history, especially when indicating the likelihood of adhesive disease and/or adjacent adnexal disease may significantly raise the level of surgical difficulty and case complexity. In less experienced surgeons these cases should be initially avoided without proctorship and consideration may be given to less complex modalities such as conventional laparoscopy or laparotomy. Once comfortable and experienced, a surgeon's patient selection can then be opened to more complex and larger pathology.

Important Differences from Multiport Robotics.

There are many important differences between robotic multiport and robotic single-site surgical platforms. There are no advanced instruments such as the Intuitive Vessel Sealer™ for use in the single-site set. The set does contain a full range of graspers, however they have no energy application available to them. As a result, with the standard set your energy comes from two instruments, a fenestrated bipolar grasper (for burning and sealing) and a monopolar hook (mainly for cutting.) Another major difference from Multiport is the loss of wristed instruments in the single-site set. In fact, only the needle driver instrument is wristed. All other single-site instruments are straight. Another major difference is that the instruments are flexible. While this maximizes triangulation, it also serves to take away from maximum instrument force and torque. This is most noticeable during suturing or "traction-counter-traction" movements. Because of these changes the single-site instruments actually cost less than the multiport instruments, which is an advantage. This cost change actually brings robotic single-site surgery closer in cost to conventional laparoscopic surgery than to multiport robotic assisted surgery [7]. Hopefully in the future these costs will continue to decline.

3. Set up

Correctly completing the set-up process is extremely important to a successful surgery, as it allows instruments to be in their proper place to allow for maximum movement. When using the Intuitive Gelport™, there will be an arrow which needs to point towards the target anatomy when placed in the abdomen. This aligns the port entries of the Gelport.

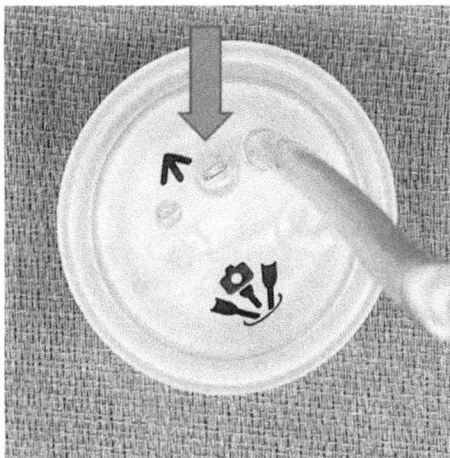

Figure 1.
Intuitive Gelport(™).

After placement in the abdomen, the ports are placed in the following sequence: The camera port is placed first in the top port site as indicated by the blue arrow (**Figure 1**).

(The camera port is placed first in the top port site as indicated by the blue arrow).

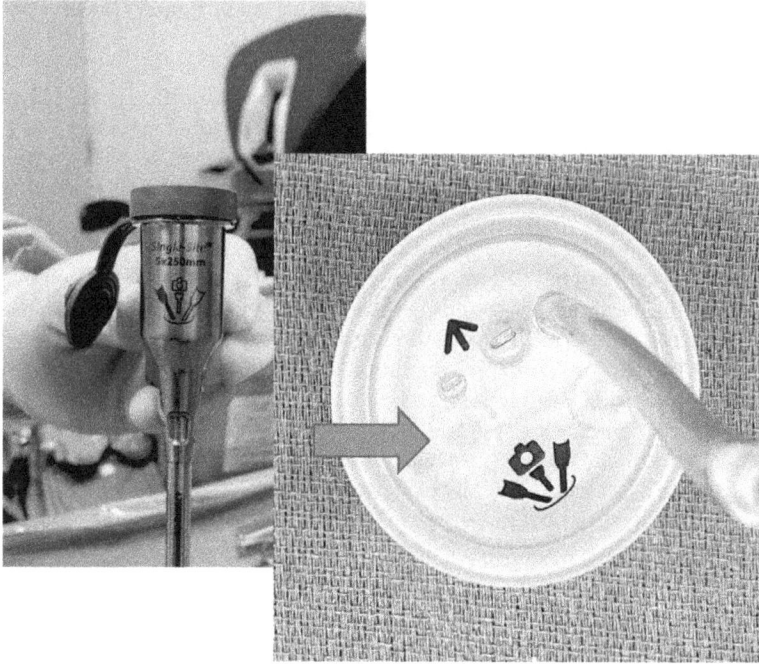

Figure 2.
The left trocar and Gelport are shown prior to insertion.

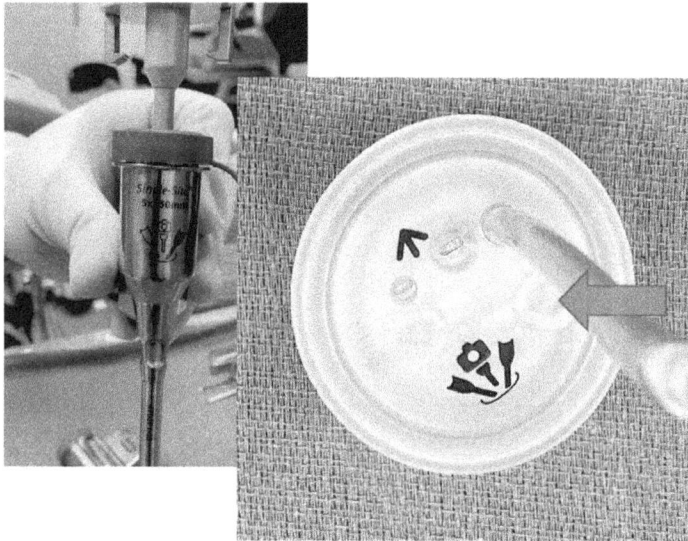

Figure 3.
The right trocar and Gelport are shown prior to insertion.

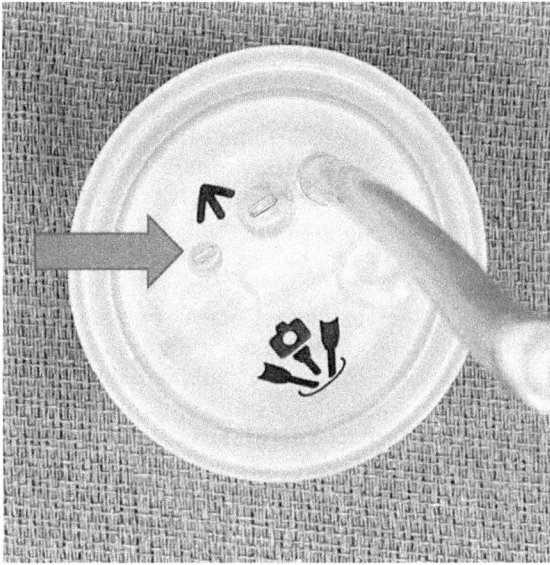

Figure 4.
Gelport is shown with the assistant port indicated by the blue arrow.

This is followed by the shaded left curved trocar (Xi system) in the left out-side port site indicated by the blue arrow, or the #2 curved trocar (Si System) (**Figure 2**).

The shaded right curved trocar is then placed in the right lateral port site indicated by the blue arrow or the #1 curved trocar (**Figure 3**).

Last, the assistant port is placed in the port site on the left side of the camera port as indicated by the blue arrow (**Figure 4**).

4. Robot positioning

Another important step is the positioning of the Da Vinci surgical system itself. The Xi system, which has better range of motion, can be angled on either right or left side facing towards the patient's hip and the overhead boom is rotated into place. If using the Si system, the robot must be positioned directly between the patient's legs leaving enough space for the bottom assistant. The right and left arms of the Si system are bent at the first joint and locked into place to allow for instrument triangulation.

5. Operating

Begin by placing your preferred uterine manipulator. At our institution we commonly use the Delineator™ from CooperSurgical™. Following this, your attention turns to the abdomen to identify the best position for the 2.5 cm incision that will be placed. This incision can be directly within the umbilicus or directly above or below the umbilicus. Typically, the lines of the umbilicus are used, and a verti-cal incision is most commonly made directly through the umbilicus. This allows for concealment of the incision line creating a superior cosmetic effect. Another common incision is a "U" incision cut either inferior or superiorly made. Great care should be taken while performing this step and again at the time of skin closure to ensure careful reconstruction. This will ensure the best cosmetic results. At times the umbilical stalk can be detached during entry. If this occurs, it should be reattached to the fascia for best cosmetic effect, preserving the depth of the umbilicus. Typically, a 2.5 cm–3 cm incision is required to install the Intuitive Gelport(™). If the incision is made too small, a visible dark, purplish ring can be seen on the skin around the umbilicus resulting from pressure necrosis. Although we have found that this usually heals over time without complication, this can simply be prevented by creating an appropriately sized incision in the first place.

Next, the fascia is identified and incised to the same length. The intuitive Gelport is then clamped at the base with long tissue forceps. Be careful not to grasp the small bronze sphere on the bottom of the port as this is part of the insufflation mechanism on the Gelport, and could be damaged by the forceps (**Figures 5** and **6**).

An army/navy retractor is then used to lift the inferior opening of the incision and the clamped gelport is inserted with downward pressure through the incision until the port is buried to the upper base. Traction and counter traction are used to perform this. Once inserted, the army/navy is again used, this time in a circular motion to sink the port into place beyond its initial ring.

Once the port is in place, gas is attached to the Gelport and insufflation begins. The single-site camera trocar is then inserted into the appropriate space in the Gelport. The trocar should be moistened with saline. Do not use gel as it will cause the trocar to slip from position during the procedure.

The patient can now be placed into Trendelenburg and the camera inserted to survey the surgical field. A 30-degree angled scope is recommended. The robot can then be moved into position and the camera docked into the trocar.

Insertion of the trocars begins with the left curved trocar first, and then the right curved trocar. While holding the port with the left hand, the right hand guides the curved trocar which starts parallel with the patient abdomen and is moved until the marked arrow passes through the Gelport. The trocar is then moved vertically and advanced to the solid line on the trocar (**Figure 7**).

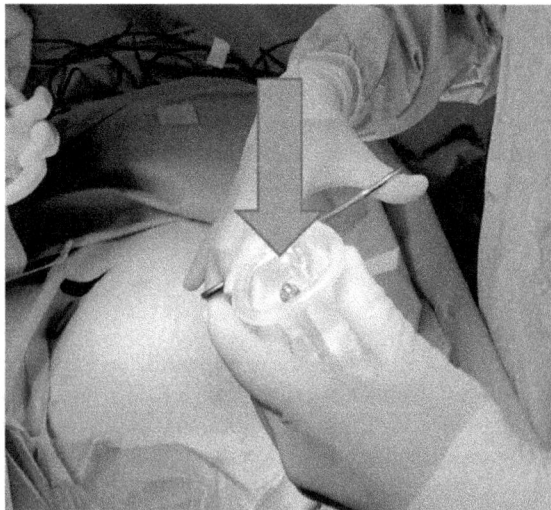

Figure 5.
A red arrow shows the small bronze sphere on the bottom of the Gelport. This is part of the insufflation mechanism on the Gelport, and could be damaged if inadvertently grasped by the forceps.

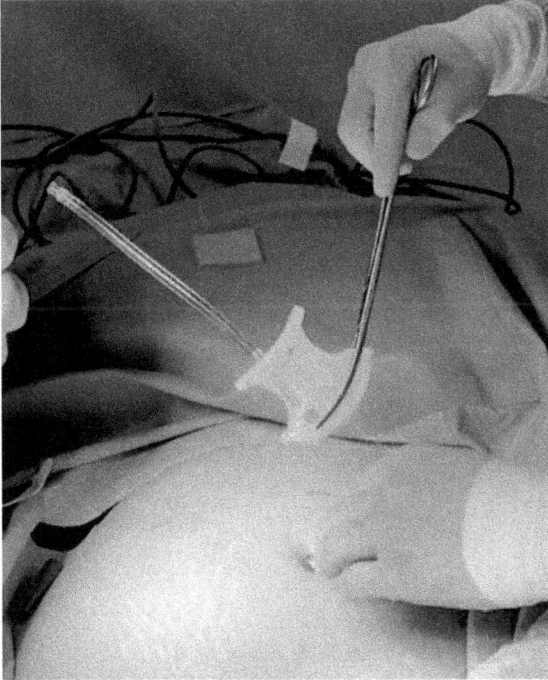

Figure 6.
Proper grasping of the base of the Gelport with forceps is shown.

At the same time the trocar tip can be seen on the screen entering the patient's right side.

Note that as the trocar passes into the abdomen it crosses over to the opposite side.

The same procedure is then repeated with the right trocar. Again, it enters from the right side and passes to the left side of the patient (**Figure 8**).

The 30-degree scope can be rotated to opposite sides to visualize the trocars safely entering the abdomen (**Figure 9**).

The camera port is then brought to a 90-degree angle, with the skin of the abdomen, and the assistant port is inserted until the pre-marked area is reached. A 5 mm or 10 mm assist port can be used. At our institution, I prefer an 8 mm AirSeal™ port. The camera is then brought back to center with the trocar tips in view. All trocars are then docked and positioned. The trocars should be clearly visible on the right and left sides of the camera view. Remember all trocars are moistened with saline prior to positioning in the Gelport. Again we do not recommend using gel to avoid slippage during the procedure.

Once the robot is docked, the left sided instrument clutch is pressed. This will reassign the right and left arms making the right internal arm now controlled by your right joystick, and the left internal arm now controlled by your left joystick. This switch allows the surgeon sitting at the console to have traditional right and left control. The instruments most commonly used for hysterectomy will be the Monopolar Hook and the Fenestrated Bipolar grasper. With the trocars crossed the monopolar hook is commonly placed in the left trocar and becomes your right arm. The fenestrated bipolar grasper is placed in the right trocar and becomes the left arm. Many authors have described constant camera and instrument movement as well as frequent clutch control as factors most associated with success [8, 9]. Constant centering of instruments allows for maximum traction and counter traction movement.

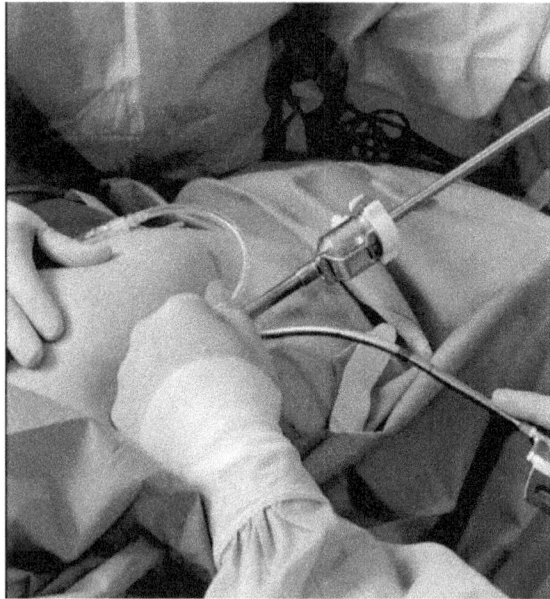

Figure 7.
The left curved trocar is inserted first, as shown in this picture.

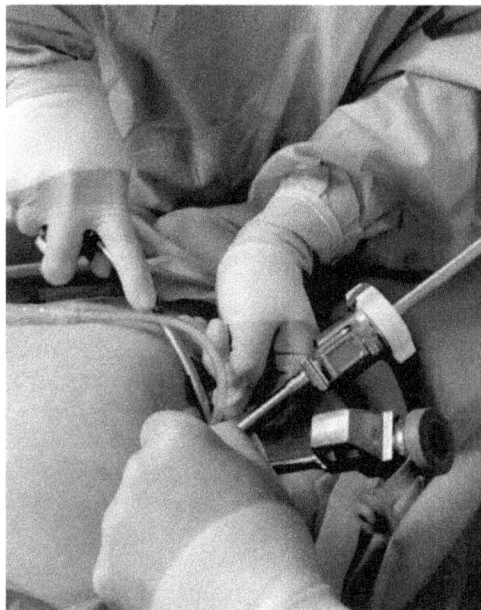

Figure 8.
A 30-degree scope is ideal for visualizing the insertion of the lateral trocars.

Another factor that plays a large role in successful robotic single-site surgery is the uterine manipulating device (and the assistant controlling it). Their strategic movements of the uterus help bring the tissue to the instruments and are crucial to procedure success [10].

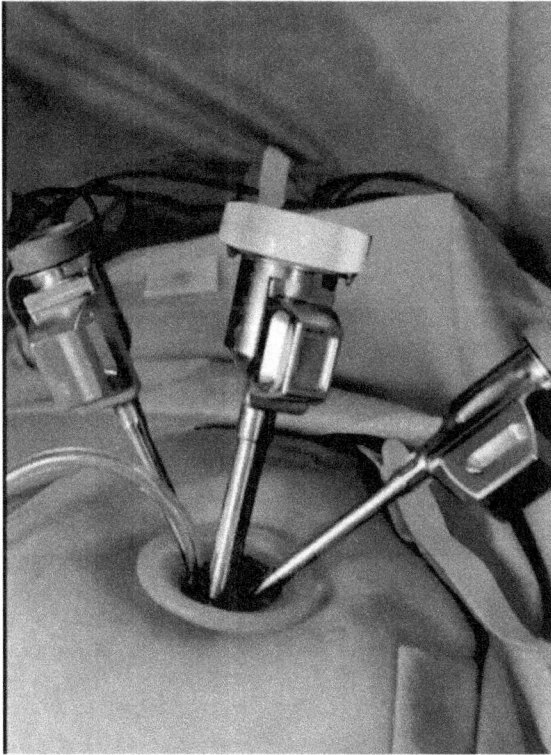

Figure 9.
Installation is complete with the camera and both trocars in position.

The initial steps in a robotic single-site hysterectomy largely depend on if the ovaries are to be removed or remain, as this will determine the plane of dissection. The round ligament is coagulated with the fenestrated Bipolar and transected with the Monopolar hook. The anterior and posterior peritoneal planes are separated with traction and counter traction and Monopolar Hook to skeletonize the uterine vasculature down to the uterine artery. A bladder flap is then created by dividing the vesico-uterine fascia, and the bladder is bluntly pushed out of the operating field. Traction and counter traction are again used for dissecting and opening the bladder flap. Once the flap is created, the ring or cup of the uterine manipulator must be identified. The colpotomy is begun in the anterior portion and is made with the hook cautery. This acts to further isolate the uterine arteries. Surgeon's preference may dictate coagulating the uterine arteries before the colotomy is made or as they are identified while creating the colpotomy. The arteries are coagulated and sealed using the fenestrated bipolar grasper and transected with the monopolar hook. The colpotomy can then be completed using the hook. Once the uterus is detached and removed, our next step will be the closure of the vaginal cuff.

Robotic single-site suturing has great advantages over laparoscopic suturing because of the availability of wristed instruments. The wristed needle driver is, in fact, the only wristed instrument in the set. When closing the vaginal cuff, the fenestrated arm can remain on the left arm to allow for grasping of the vaginal cuff. The monopolar hook is replaced with the wristed needle driver. The wristed single-site needle driver's movements are slightly more encumbered in comparison to the multiport version, however it is still wristed and allows for increased articulation for driving a needle. Another difference is the loss of strength or torque in using the single-site needle driver due to its curved flexible nature. My preferred suture and needle is a barbed 2.0 trimethylene carbonate suture on a P14 reverse cutting needle V-Loc™. Many authors have recommended this system for cuff closure when performing a robotic single-site hysterectomy [11]. This allows for an easier drive of the needle through the cuff for suturing. Another way to help with instrument torque or force if having trouble driving the needle, is to advance the trocars slightly inward to decrease the flexibility of the instruments. In my experience, mastery of traction and counter traction are the keys to successful closure. The needle is small enough to pass through the 8 mm air seal port for entry and removal. I recommend 1–2 redundant throws of the V-Loc™ stitch device in order to secure the suture line after completing the vaginal closure.

6. Closing the fascia

Once the surgery has been safely completed, remove all trocars so that only the camera and assistant trocars remain and evacuate the gas. Next, grasp the gel port and place a lap sponge over the Gelport to prevent splashing and gently remove the port. To close the fascial opening, I recommend grasping the fascial edge with a kocher clamp and securing each edge with a figure-of-eight stitch using a 0 vicryl on a UR6 needle, and then holding the tissue with hemostat clamps. Next, with an army/navy, I recommend grasping the lateral edges and displacing them outward and then upward using the hemostats. This will bring the fascia away from the underlying bowel. Finally, finish closing the fascia with several more figure-of-eight sutures. Generally, approximately 4–5 figure-of-eight sutures are needed to complete the closure. Lastly, I recommend reapproximating the subcutaneous tissues with 3–0 vicryl and performing skin closure with 4–0 monocryl followed by Dermabond™ adhesive.

7. Special considerations

There are surgical considerations when performing robotic single-site laparoscopic surgery.

Visually the surgeon will be operating from the midline or a slightly off center position. In these situations, a 30-degree scope can be very helpful. Camera movements and instrument movements are all occurring in a very confined space within the center of the screen. Surgical instruments cannot cross or move to as far as their multiport versions can. They cannot reach opposite ends of the screen. As the instruments follow camera movement, camera clutching and instrument movements are frequently needed in order to move around the surgical field and operate safely and effectively. Instrument tips are typically working side by side.

In addition, the surgical assistant controlling the assistant port may have a challenging task. They will have limited freedom of movement and need to keep their instrument in the view of the camera at all times. The assistant must carefully control the movement of their instrument, such as a suction irrigator or a grasper. One technique to give the accessory port some additional freedom is to occasionally pull back on the camera and attempt to visualize the operative area from under the assistant's instrument. This technique resembles diving downward in practice. Generally, this will create some freedom of operation to avoid collision with your assistant's instrument. Care and vigilance must be taken, however, because too much movement may still move the assistant which can lead to unintended tissue trauma. As a result, constant coordination between the movements of the surgeon and the surgical assistant is critical for safe, effective surgery.

If during a robotic single-site case, the surgeon encounters complex pathology and the case becomes too difficult to complete through single-site technique, the surgeon then has several options. The operator is able to utilize the 4th arm of the DaVinci robot and add an extra lateral single multiport trocar. This allows for utilization of an extra multiport surgical arm and the use of a full wristed surgical instrument such as a Vessel Sealer or Monopolar Scissors. This conversion makes it a robotic single-site plus one surgery. If the surgeon continues to have difficulty safely completing the surgery, then the robotic single-site surgery can be fully converted to traditional robotic multiport by removing the curved trocars and adding both right and left lateral abdominal multiport trocars. The gelport with the camera trocar can remain along with the assistant port or the assistant port can be moved to a more traditional site. This allows the surgery to remain a minimally invasive approach before needing to convert to laparotomy.

Once the surgeon operates consistently and becomes more comfortable and confident another port option is the GelPoint™ or GelPoint Mini™ from Applied Medical. The GelPoint and Gelpoint mini allows for a smaller 2.0–2.5 cm incision and an increased range of motion with your single-site instruments. We do not recommend starting single site training with these ports because of the increased range of the instruments can lead to sudden slippage. This can lead to uncontrolled movements and possible surgical complications. Instrument control must be mastered prior to attempting these modifications. Also, the gel interface of the Gelpoint™ is known to be more prone to leaking gas due to tearing than it's Gelport™ counterpart. To negate this loss of gas, an AirSeal™ port can be used to hold the pneumoperitoneum (**Table 2**).

Advantages	Disadvantages
High Definition 3D immersed vision console	The loss of instrument strength and torque
Complete instrument and camera control	Loss of wristed instruments
Superior instrument movement	Limited range of motion
No instrument clashing	Surgical assist movements are limited
Superior cosmetic incision	
Suturing is made easier	
Port incision allows for large tissue extraction	
Competitive surgical cost	

Table 2.
Advantages and disadvantages of single port robotic surgery.

8. In conclusion

Minimally invasive surgery continues to evolve providing dedicated surgeons with the instruments and confidence to bring less invasive procedures to patients. I have enjoyed learning and mastering these skills over the years. I have experienced great patient satisfaction as well and personal satisfaction in my surgical journey. I look forward along with many of my colleagues to the future and the continued advancements of minimally invasive surgery and robotics.

Author details

Rene I. Luna
Women's Robotic Surgery, Renaissance Women's Hospital, Institute for Robotic
Surgery, University of Texas Rio Grande Valley, McAllen, Texas, USA

*Address all correspondence to: drlunaobgyn@gmail.com

IntechOpen

References

[1] Tracy CR, Raman JD, Cadeddu JA, Rane A. Laparoendoscopic single-site surgery in urology: where have we been and where are we heading? Nat Clin Pract Urol. 2008;5:561-8.

[2] Fanfani F, Fagotti A, Rossitto C, Gagliardi ML, Ercoli A, Gallotta V, Alletti SG, Monterossi G, Turco LC, Scambia G. Laparoscopic, minilaparoscopic and single-port hysterectomy: perioperative outcomes. Surgical endoscopy. 2012 Dec 1;26(12):3592-6.

[3] Jung YW, Kim YT, Lee DW, Im Hwang Y, Nam EJ, Kim JH, Kim SW. The feasibility of scarless single-port transumbilical total laparoscopic hysterectomy: initial clinical experience. Surgical endoscopy. 2010 Jul 1;24(7):1686-92.

[4] Lux MM, Marshall M, Erturk E, Joseph JV. Ergonomic evaluation and guidelines for use of the daVinci Robot system. Journal of endourology. 2010 Mar 1;24(3):371-5.

[5] Angioni S, Pontis A, Pisanu A, et al. Single-port access subtotal laparoscopic hysterectomy: a prospective case-control study. J Minim Invasive. 2015;22:809-12.

[6] American College of Obstetricians and Gynecologists. Choosing the route of hysterectomy for benign disease. ACOG Committee Opinion No. 444. Obstetrics and Gynecology. 2009;114(5):1156-8.

[7] Arghami A, Dy BM, Bingener J, Osborn J, Richards ML. Single-port robotic-assisted adrenalectomy: feasibility, safety, and cost-effectiveness. JSLS: Journal of the Society of Laparoendoscopic Surgeons. 2015 Jan;19(1).

[8] Palep JH. Robotic assisted minimally invasive surgery. Journal of minimal access surgery. 2009 Jan;5(1):1.

[9] Stegemann AP, Ahmed K, Syed JR, Rehman S, Ghani K, Autorino R, Sharif M, Rao A, Shi Y, Wilding GE, Hassett JM. Fundamental skills of robotic surgery: a multi-institutional randomized controlled trial for validation of a simulation-based curriculum. Urology. 2013 Apr 1;81(4):767-74.

[10] Senapati S, Advincula AP. Surgical techniques: robot-assisted laparoscopic myomectomy with the da Vinci® surgical system. Journal of Robotic Surgery. 2007 Mar 1;1(1):69.

[11] Cong L, Li C, Wei B, Zhan L, Wang W, Xu Y. V-Loc™ 180 suture in total laparoscopic hysterectomy: a retrospective study comparing Polysorb to barbed suture used for vaginal cuff closure. European Journal of Obstetrics & Gynecology and Reproductive Biology. 2016 Dec 1;207:18-22.

Chapter 6

Utility of Robotic Assisted and Single Site Laparoscopy to Gynecologic Oncology

Conor J. Corcoran and Stephen H. Bush II

Abstract

Single site laparoscopy, while in its infancy, is being explored for potential areas of application within the realm of gynecology. Gynecologic Oncology is a field with high potential benefit from the single site technique. It boasts many practical and theoretical surgical improvements, such as facilitated specimen removal, which are elaborated further in this chapter. While much more research is needed, there are exciting and uniquely useful utilities of Laparo-endoscopic Single-site Surgery (LESS) in gynecology oncology.

Keywords: Gynecology Oncology, minimally invasive surgery, cancer, mini-laparotomy, surgical staging

1. Introduction

Historically, gynecologic oncology has been dominated by laparotomy for peritoneal access, and this has carried partially even into the era of minimally invasive surgery [1]. There were good reasons for initial concern regarding laparoscopy, including port site metastasis, intact specimen removal, and technical complications of staging. Many would credit the hallmark LAP2 trial [2] with forever changing the face of gynecologic oncology, as it was the first high powered study to demonstrate laparoscopy to be comparable to laparotomy in gynecologic oncology procedures. This, combined with the already known advantages of minimally invasive surgery over classic laparotomy, launched the advent of laparoscopy in gynecologic oncology, in the opinion of many. The advantages were seen initially in the treatment of uterine cancer [3]. Many feel the extrapolation of this data was the impetus that eventually led to the saturation of minimally invasive surgery in the treatment of all other gynecologic malignant processes. With decreased length of stay, lower hernia rates, improved cosmesis, and lower infection rate, laparoscopy quickly became the preferred surgical methodology across gynecologic oncology. Gynecologic oncology has since contributed countless minimally invasive techniques since the LAP2 trial. Most notably, gynecologic oncologists were among the first to utilize and publish on single site laparoscopy [4–7].

Single site laparoscopic surgery provides many of the same potential improvements in cosmesis as benign gynecology, but also may hold the critical benefit of facilitated intact specimen extraction [8]. Removal of the intact specimen is generally a critical aspect of oncologic surgery, as attempting to avoid tumor spillage into body cavities is a critical concept in the treatment of malignancy [9]. This fulfills

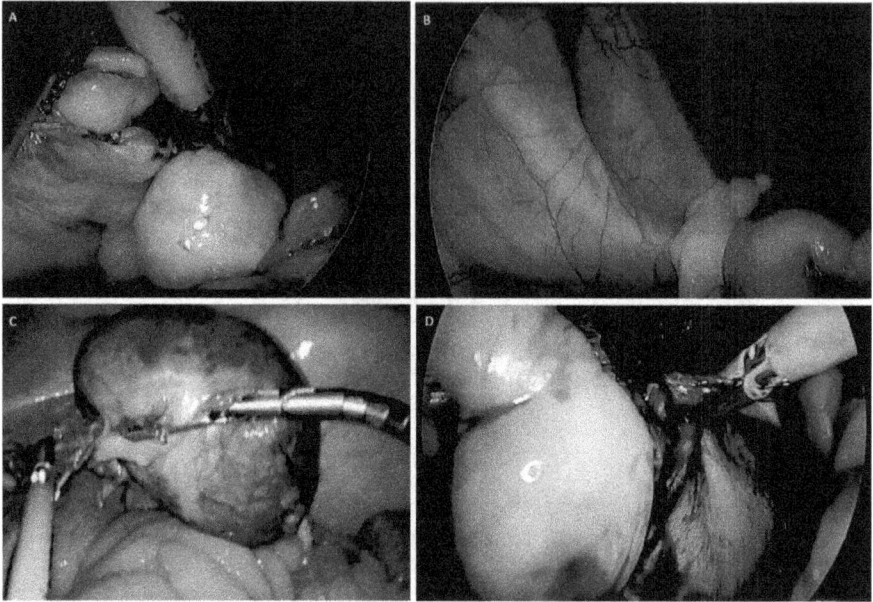

Figure 1.
(A) Completion of Salpingectomy vNTOES single site (B) Single site vNOTES visualization of the ureter. (C) Large adnexal mass liberated during laparoscopic single site surgery. (D) Uterine artery ligation and cauterization during vNOTES.

what many authors refer to as the so-called "Goldilocks" concept of specimen removal [10], allowing the surgical oncologist to laparoscopically remove larger organ systems, a feat which which would have required laparotomy previously. Multiple methods of large specimen extraction in standard laparoscopy have been described, ranging from mini-laparotomy [11, 12] and nonstandard incisions [13], to incisional extension. While useful techniques, these are less studied in malignant processes and their long term sequelae are less elucidated. Therein, many would consider that Laparoendoscopic Single-site Surgery (LESS) techniques have great merit and promise in Gynecologic Oncology (**Figure 1**).

2. Applications for gynecologic oncology

The majority of studies done to date in gynecology oncologic are case series or longitudinal studies done at major facilities in the United States, United Kingdom, and China. The first reports of use and feasibility highlighted the expected benefits of standard laparoscopy with the improvement of single incision cosmesis, decreased blood loss, and decreased pain. Decreased pain was the most consistent finding among early publications, which was noted in a Cochrane review of LESS in benign and oncologic gynecology [14]. Here we will outline specific advantages of the single-site technique and other considerations for specific gynecologic malignant processes.

2.1 Uterine cancers

The majority of LESS procedures have been performed for hysterectomy in uterine cancers, (mirroring the LAP2 trial [2]) and for risk-reducing salpingecto-mies. These have included, in some studies, lymphadenectomy for cancer staging purposes [15]. Given the literature available, there are many potential benefits offered by LESS techniques, including: preventing peritoneal tumor spillage, tissue preservation for pathologic analysis, and facilitation of extraction.

LESS requires more time to master for advanced retroperitoneal dissection and lymphadenectomies, but a surgeon adept at traditional laparoscopic surgery can overcome these challenges and master these techniques relatively quickly. Patient selection is also of the utmost importance, as obesity is a well known major risk factor for endometrial cancer, and this excess adiposity can increase the difficulty of the already complex LESS procedure.

In 2012 a publication from Memorial Sloan Kettering Cancer Center on sentinel node biopsy in endometrial cancer, it was suggested to change the standard practice in the United States to a sentinel node algorithm rather than comprehensive lymphadenectomy in most patients with endometrial adenocarcinoma [16]. Their algorithm suggested: (1) peritoneal evaluation thorough inspection and washing, (2) retroperitoneal evaluation with excision of all mapped or suspicious nodes, (3) side specific lymph node dissection in case of no mapping into a hemi-pelvis, (4) para-aortic node dissection performed at the discretion of the attending surgeon [12].

Sentinel node biopsy and mapping was gained acceptance as the standard of care for endometrial cancer. This comes after multiple publications such as the FIRES trial which paved the way for the NCCN guidelines suggesting LESS techniques may be adopted more easily, given the need for less extensive dissection and ease at transition to a multiport procedure when needed [17].

A new subfield of LESS, vaginal natural orifice transluminal endoscopic surgery (vNOTES) is emerging in the field of gynecologic surgery. While the vast majority of investigation of vNOTES has been in benign gynecology, there are recent documented applications for oncologic purposes, specifically for early stage endometrial cancer (**Figure 2**).

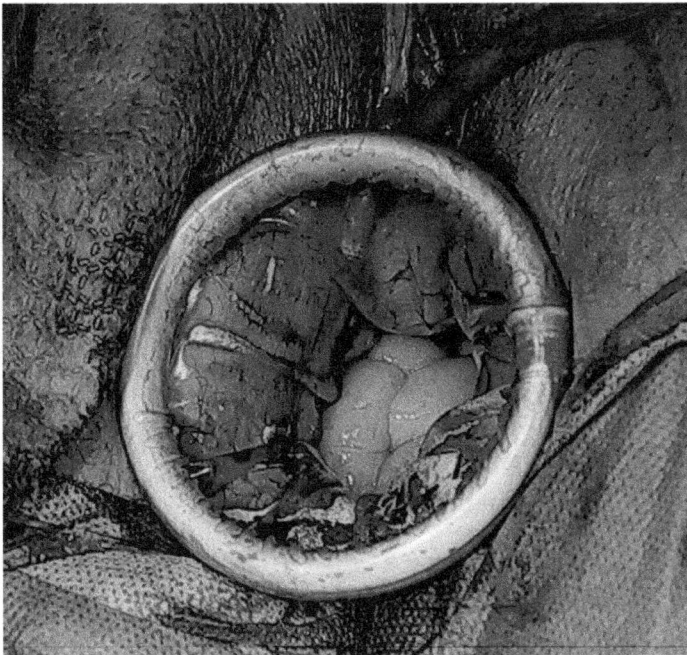

Figure 2.
Single site wound retractor applied to the vagina status post vaginal hysterectomy, accessing the peritoneum for vNOTES procedure.

2.2 Cervical cancers

Interestingly, there were successful publications on using single-site for radical hysterectomy for early stage cervical cancers. The theoretical benefits of LESS were similar to the general benefits mentioned previously. Unfortunately, a landmark 2018 study performed by Ramirez et al., (the LACC trial,) [18] demonstrated a decrease in overall and disease-free survival with laparoscopic radical hysterectomies for early cervical cancers. As a result, laparoscopic radical hysterectomies have become rare in practice [19]. Therefore, until confounding literature published, many gynecologic oncologists feel the utility of LESS for radical hysterectomy is limited and maybe more of an interesting historical footnote than a viable procedure.

2.3 Ovarian cancer

While it is widely considered that advanced ovarian cancers may still be best managed via laparotomy, laparoscopy and robot assisted laparoscopy is still routinely utilized in early stage ovarian cancers. Complete staging is imperative for all ovarian malignancies. The protocol for assessing these early ovarian cancers includes: lymph node dissection, peritoneal biopsies, and omentectomy. These measures allow for peritoneal sampling which allows for improved detection of micro-metastatic disease, which, in turn, optimizes adjuvant chemotherapeutic selection and prognosis for patients.

Perhaps the greatest area of potential use in Gynecologic Oncology for LESS techniques would be adnexal masses. When the uterus is left in situ in traditional laparoscopic surgery retrieval of a large adnexal mass can be very frustrating. A 10 or 12 mm incision is often not large enough for removal of a large specimen. As a result, this scenario requires an incision to be extended, (including fascial extension) and creates a risk of injury to the bowel or other structures, as well as a risk of spillage from the isolating bag. LESS techniques in general will require a 2-3 cm umbilical incision but this can be made larger for certain clinical scenarios. Making the incision in a natural defect such as the umbilicus can yield excellent cosmetic results when a larger incision for extraction is required [20].

For a suspicious mass large extraction bags are available in sizes up to 17 cm. These vary in size and shape and are available from various manufacturers. They can be deployed intraperitoneally and the mass can be brought out through the umbilical incision, or if necessary, drained while contained. If a frozen section

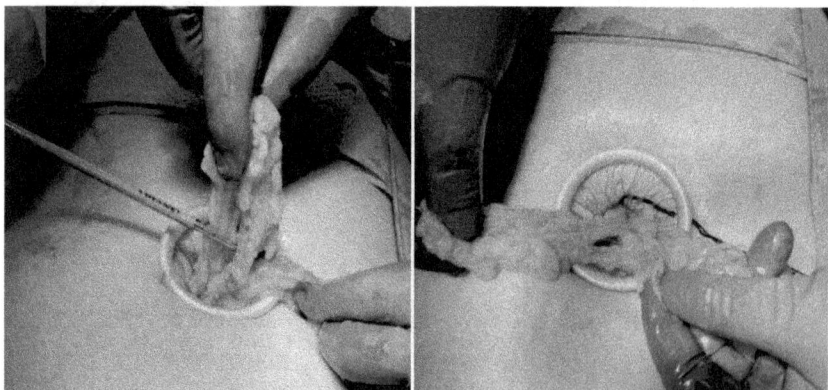

Figure 3.
Omentectomy at the time of minimally invasive removal of suspicious ovarian cyst.

is obtained and this reveals a borderline or ovarian malignancy, the surgeon may feel an infracolic omentectomy is indicated. Generally, the LESS port provides an incision large enough to deliver omentum intact and large enough to perform a relatively easy and quick infracolic omentectomy using whatever laparoscopic energy device has already been used. This technique is similar to previous described techniques of omentectomy performed through a miniature laparotomy (**Figure 3**).

For the very large benign appearing mass with normal tumor markers in a young patient, a LESS approach through the umbilicus can facilitate contained drainage. After placing the LESS port of choice the mass can be visualized before insufflation. One technique is to place two purse string sutures of 3-0 monofilament suture into the mass concentric to each other. A small hole is then made and the suction aspirator inserted with the inner stitch tied to contain leakage. Once the mass is decompressed the suction aspirator is removed, and the outer stitch can be tied to prevent any further spillage. The decompressed mass is then removed laparoscopically. The slightly large incision in the umbilicus usually allows for easy removal.

It is important to note that the above techniques for adnexal mass removal are not appropriate for all patients. For any patients in which a malignancy is suspected, great care must be taken to avoid any technique that introduces the risk of spilling malignant cells in the abdominal cavity, effectively working to spread the lesion. For patients with a low suspicion of malignancy, however, we feel that the technique is a welcome addition to the armamentarium of the gynecologic surgeon. We welcome further research, including case studies and described techniques. This will serve to further develop the minimally invasive literature as well as to stimulate ideas for new clinical trial protocols.

2.4 Robotic applications

A number of studies have been performed in the realm of benign gynecology with robotic LESS with varied success. Few, however, have been published specifically on oncologic robotic surgery. The most notable of these demonstrated the feasibility of robotic single-site [21]. The benefits and pitfalls of robotic single-site surgery are similar to benign gynecology as previously discussed in this text [22].

3. Limitations and considerations

Despite the various sources listed in this chapter and the multitude of studies on LESS for gynecologic oncology, there is an overall lack of data on the topic given its relatively new emergence. With only a decade passing since first recorded data in this topic, more research will need done before long-term conclusions can be drawn. To date, the longest single study follow up our authors could find was 3 years [23, 24].

Perhaps more than any other adverse outcome, there is evidence that LESS techniques may hold a higher hernia rate than previously expected [1, 13–16]. One study by Multon et al. demonstrated that hernia rates within 1 year are similar to standard laparoscopy (5.5%), 3 year follow up seemed to indicate a significant increase in hernia rates as high as 23% [1]. As a result, several authors have stated that it would appear the increased incision size for LESS may have a greater effect on incisional hernia than previously thought [25, 26].

The technical difficulties of LESS techniques are identical to the benign gynecologic applications of the surgical method, including loss of triangulation, arm clashing, and surgeon comfort [27]. With training, time, and improving surgical instruments, these limitations may be overcome.

4. Conclusion

LESS appears to be a viable, safe alternative to standard laparoscopy for most gynecologic oncology procedures. While more research is needed and is ongoing, it is the hope of the authors that more will endeavor and utilize single-site techniques for oncologic cases.

Author details

Conor J. Corcoran[1] and Stephen H. Bush II [1,2*]

1 Charleston Area Medical Center, USA

2 West Virginia University School of Medicine Charleston Division, USA

*Address all correspondence to: sbush1@gmail.com

IntechOpen

References

[1] Moulton, L et al. Single-port laparoscopy in gynecologic oncology: seven years of experience at a single institution. Am J Obstet Gynecol. 2017;217(5):610.e1-610.e.8.

[2] Walker, JL et al. Laparoscopy compared with laparotomy for comprehensive surgical staging of uterine cancer: Gynecologic Oncology Group study LAP2. J Clin Oncol. 2009;27:5331-5336.

[3] Cho YH, Kim DY, Kim JH, Kim YM, Kim YT, Nam JH. Laparoscopic management of early uterine cancer: 10-year experience in Asan Medical Center. Gynecologic oncology. 2007 Sep 1;106(3):585-90.

[4] Pontis, A et al. Review and meta-analysis of prospective randomized controlled trials (RCTs) comparing laparo-endoscopic single site and multiport laparoscopy in gynecologic operative procedures. Arch Gynecol Obstet. 2016;294:567-577.

[5] Escobar, PF et al. Single-port laparoscopic pelvic and para-aortic lymph node sampling or lymphadenectomy: development of a technique and instrumentation. Int J Gynecol Cancer. 2010;20:1268-1273.

[6] Escobar, PF et al. Single-port risk-reducing salpingo-oophorectomy with and without hysterectomy: surgical outcomes and learning curve analysis. Gynecol Oncol. 2010;119:43-47.

[7] Single-port vs multiport laparoscopic hysterectomy: a meta-analysis of randomized controlled trials. J Minim Invasive Gynecol. 2016;23:1049-1056.

[8] Fader, AN & Escobar, PF. Laparoscopic single-site surgery (LESS) in gynecologic oncology: Technique and initial report.

[9] Richardson H. Goldilocks Mastectomy 24. Oncoplastic Breast Surgery Techniques for the General Surgeon. 2020 May 22:413.

[10] Matanes E, Lauterbach R, Boulus S, Amit A, Lowenstein L. Robotic laparoendoscopic single-site surgery in gynecology: a systematic review. European Journal of Obstetrics & Gynecology and Reproductive Biology. 2018 Dec 1;231:1-7.

[11] Kato, K. *et al.* 2017. "Extraction of a specimen through an umbilical zigzag incision during laparoscopic surgery for endometrial cancer". Kato et al. World Journal of Surgical Oncology (2017) 15:110. DOI 10.1186/s12957-017-1180-x.

[12] P. B. Panici, M. A. Zullo, R. Angioli, and L. Muzii, "Minilaparotomy hysterectomy. A valid option for the treatment of benign uterine pathologies," *European Journal of Obstetrics Gynecology and Reproductive Biology*, vol. 119, no. 2, pp. 228-231, 2005.

[13] Buckley III, FP et al. Influencing factors for port-site hernias after single-incision laparoscopy. Hernia. 2016;20:729-733.

[14] Sasada T, Murakami S, Kataoka T, Ohara M, Ozaki S, Okada M, Ohdan H. Memorial Sloan-Kettering Cancer Center Nomogram to predict the risk of non-sentinel lymph node metastasis in Japanese breast cancer patients. Surgery today. 2012 Mar;42(3):245-9.

[15] Fagotti, A. et al. First 100 early endometrial cancer cases treated with Laparoendoscopic single-site surgery: a multicentric retrospective study. Am J Obstet Gynecol. 2012;206:353.e.1-353.e.6.

[16] Jennings, AJ et al. The feasibility and safety of adopting single-incision

laparoscopic surgery into gynecologic oncology practice. J Minim Invasive Gynecol. 2016; 23:358-363.

[17] Tergas AI & Fader, AN. Laparoendoscopic single-site surgery (LESS) radical hysterectomy for the treatment of early stage cervical cancer. Gynecol Oncol 2013; 129:241-243.

[18] Ramirez PT, Frumovitz M, Pareja R, Lopez A, Vieira MA, Ribeiro R. Phase III randomized trial of laparoscopic or robotic versus abdominal radical hysterectomy in patients with early-stage cervical cancer: LACC Trial. Gynecologic Oncology. 2018 Jun 1;149:245.

[19] Boruta, DM et al. Laparoendoscopic single-site radical hysterectomy with pelvic lymphadenectomy: Initial multi-institutional experience for treatment of invasive cervical cancer. J Minim Invasive Gynecol. 2014;21:394-398.

[20] Gunderson, CC et al. The risk of umbilical hernia and other complications with laparoendoscopic single-site surgery. J Minim Invasive Gynecol. 2012;19:40-45.

[21] Agaba, EA et al. Incidence of port-site incisional hernia after single-incision laparoscopic surgery. JSLS. 2014;18:204-210.

[22] Antoniou, SA et al. Single-incision laparoscopic surgery through the umbilicus is associated with a higher incidence of trocar-site hernia that conventional laparoscopy: a meta-analysis of randomized controlled trials. Hernia. 2016;20:1-10.

[23] P. Royo, J. L. Alcázar, M. García-Manero, B. Olartecoechea, and G. López-García, "The value of minilaparotomy for total hysterectomy for benign uterine disease: a comparative study with conventional Pfannenstiel and laparoscopic approaches," *International Archives of Medicine*, vol. 2, article 11, 2009.

[24] Ramirez, P. *et al.* "Minimally invasive versus abdominal radical hysterectomy for Cervical Cancer". New England Journal of Medicine, 2018; 379:1895-1904.

[25] Nam, E. *et al.* "Robotic Single-port transumbilical total hysterectomy: a pilot study". J Gynecol Oncol. 2011 Jun;22(2):120-126.

[26] Barlin JN, Khoury-Collado F, Kim CH, et al. The importance of applying a sentinel lymph node mapping algorithm in endometrial cancer staging: beyond removal of blue nodes. *Gynecol Oncol*. 2012;125(3):531-535.

[27] Rossi, E.C. *et al.* A comparison of sentinel lymph node biopsy to lymphadenectomy for endometrial cancer staging (FIRES trial): a multicentre, prospective, cohort study. *Th Lancet Oncology* 2017. 18(3);384-392.

Vaginal Natural Orifice Transluminal Endoscopic Surgery for Gynecologic and Gynecologic Oncology Procedures

Alexander F. Burnett and Martha O. Rojo

Abstract

Vaginal Natural Orifice Transluminal Endoscopic Surgery (vNOTES) is an exciting new procedure that combines the best of laparoscopic and transvaginal surgery. The skills of a laparoscopic surgeon are applied to this approach which offers several advantages over traditional laparoscopy. First, the recovery of a vaginal procedure is shorter and less painful. Second, there is no abdominal incision which avoids potential for wound infection, herniation, pain and unsightly scarring. Third, the surgeon is seated with more comfortable ergonomics than traditional laparoscopy. Fourth, the blood supply is controlled very early in the procedure reducing overall blood loss. Fifth, the specimen for removal is quite close to the operator which enables less crossing of instruments and allows larger scopes with better illumination to be used. Finally, where traditional laparoscopy progresses to a smaller and smaller surgical area as the operation proceeds deeper into the pelvis, vNOTES is continually moving out of the pelvis with greater room for specimen manipulation and visualization. Advantages over traditional transvaginal surgery include the ability to examine the entire abdomen, the safety of direct visualization of the pedicles for adnexal removal, and the ability to perform abdominal procedures including lymph node removal, omentectomy, appendectomy, and biopsies not previously available to the vaginal approach.

Keywords: vNOTES, minimally invasive surgery

1. Introduction

Vaginal Natural Orifice Transluminal Endoscopic Surgery (vNOTES) incorporates a number of different techniques and strategies to permit minimally invasive surgery through the natural orifice of the vagina. It is a hybridization of laparoscopic and transvaginal approaches with the advantages of each. While some of the earliest endoscopic techniques were performed through the posterior vagina and referred to as culdoscopy, only since the adaptation of multi-port single-incision laparoscopy to a transvaginal approach has the full value of this technique begun to be appreciated. Almost any laparoscopic procedure can now be performed transvaginally which can significantly reduce patients' postoperative discomfort, time to recovery, length of hospitalization, and without visible scar.

2. History of the technique

The use of endoscopic procedures to visualize the abdomen is over 100 years old. Visualization of the pelvis through the vagina was developed by Decker who first reported the procedure in 1944 [1]. The term culdoscopy was used to describe placement of a scope into the posterior cul-de-sac with the patient in knee-chest position. This was originally used for diagnostic purposes but later modified for treatment of ovarian conditions, ectopic pregnancy and tubal ligation. However, the technique was never utilized by a wide audience of gynecologists, and abdominal and traditional transvaginal procedures continued to dominate the field. In the 1990s as fiber-optic cameras and improved instrumentation developed, abdominal laparoscopy came into vogue and has since exploded as a dominant method of performing gynecologic surgery along with its more recent counterpart, robotic surgery. Laparoscopy has replaced a large percentage of abdominal procedures permitting faster recovery, less pain, and better cosmetics for our patients. Unfortunately, as laparoscopic techniques and instrumentation continued to improve, the percent of hysterectomies performed transvaginally diminished. For example, the percent of hysterectomies performed vaginally dropped from 25% in 1998 to 17% in 2010 and continues to fall [2]. This despite the recommendation by the American College of Obstetricians and Gynecologists [3] and the AAGL [4] that transvaginal hysterectomy is the preferred method for benign gynecological disease as the optimum approach for patient safety and recovery. Younger gynecologists in academic and community settings are performing fewer transvaginal techniques. As a consequence, they are less likely to train resident physicians in transvaginal surgery.

The earliest utilization of a vNOTES approach was for general surgery procedures such as cholecystectomy and appendectomy [5]. In Asia in 2012, Ahn reported on the use of the single-port placed into the posterior vagina to remove the adnexa [6]. At the same time, the first series of vNOTES hysterectomies was published [7]. These authors utilized an Alexis retractor (Applied Medical, Rancho Santa Margarita, CA) placed into the anterior and posterior cul-de-sac with a surgical glove attached on the outer ring through which the glove fingers were used as laparoscopic ports. In Europe in 2013 Jan Baekelandt adapted the GelPoint device (Applied Medical, Rancho Santa Margarita, CA) to the transvaginal approach and has been the major developer and promoter of vNOTES surgery in the West [8, 9]. The GelPoint has the advantage of ease of set up, better ergonomics, and simplicity in specimen removal over a glove fastened to an Alexis. A group of American gynecologists (including the author of this chapter) trained with Dr. Baekelandt beginning in 2017 and brought the technique to the United States. To date, this core of vNOTES surgeons has trained approximately 100 gynecologists in this country. In 2019, a port specifically created for vNOTES (VPath, Applied Medical, Rancho Santa Margarita, CA) was developed and approved by the FDA.

3. Why perform vNOTES?

VNOTES takes advantage of the laparoscopic expertise of today's surgeons and brings it to a transvaginal platform. This combines the best of vaginal and laparoscopic surgery. The surgeon has the visualization, instrumentation and panoramic abdominal perspective of laparoscopy combined with the reduced morbidity, rapid recovery and cosmesis of vaginal surgery. The majority of vNOTES procedures can be performed as an outpatient procedure and require minimal postoperative pain medication. Most patients fully recover within two weeks of surgery, although vaginal rest continues as with any hysterectomy.

For the surgeon, the distance to the operative field is closer than with abdominal laparoscopy which translates in less collision of the instruments and permits larger scopes to be used with improved visualization. As opposed to abdominal laparoscopy where one works farther and farther down to the apex of a cone-shaped pelvis, vNOTES is constantly moving the uterus in a cephalad manner where there is more room to maneuver safely. This can be particularly advantageous with large myomatous uteri which can be manipulated farther into the abdomen as the case progresses. In addition, the major blood supply to the uterus is taken very early from a vNOTES approach which can significantly reduce blood loss. In patients with extensive adhesions from prior upper and mid abdominal surgery, vNOTES can avoid these adhesions altogether. The majority of surgeons perform this procedure while they and their assistants are seated and the ergonomics are far improved with minimal muscle strain over standard laparoscopy. This procedure is well adapted to the morbidly obese patient and can overcome surgical difficulties with standard laparoscopy including long distance to the pelvic organs, torque from traversing instruments through thick abdominal wall, and challenge of choosing appropriate port placement sites. The obese patient has the most to gain by avoidance of abdominal incisions and rapid recovery.

To date there has been one randomized trial comparing vNOTES hysterectomy with laparoscopic hysterectomy as an outpatient procedure. In this trial 70 women with benign indications for hysterectomy were randomized to either standard four incision laparoscopy for removal of the uterus or received four skin incisions without cutting through the fascia and had a vNOTES procedure [10, 11]. This permitted blinding for the patients and the investigators to which technique had occurred. There were no conversions in the study. The mean operative time for vNOTES was shorter than laparoscopy (41 minutes versus 75 minutes). More women left the hospital within 12 hours after vNOTES (77% versus 43%). Overall hospital stay was shorter for vNOTES and overall use of analgesics during the first seven days after surgery was less in the vNOTES group (eight versus 14 units). The vNOTES group also reported significantly lower Visual Analog Scores (VAS) for pain. There were also significantly fewer postoperative complications in women treated by vNOTES (9% versus 37%). In this elegant study, the outcome parameters clearly favored vNOTES over total laparoscopic hysterectomy.

4. Technique

vNOTES begins similar to a transvaginal hysterectomy. A circumferential incision is made in the cervix down to the level of the pubo-cervical fascia. The anterior and posterior aspects of the vaginal mucosa are dissected away from the cervix to gain access to the anterior and posterior cul-de-sacs. These spaces are entered, the uterosacral ligaments are clamped, cut and ligated. These pedicles may later be incorporated into cuff closure for vault support. An Alexis retractor is placed into the anterior and posterior space. The outer ring of the Alexis either has the cap attached or a glove attached depending on which one is available. The patient is placed in 20° Trendelenburg position and insufflation of the abdomen is performed. In general lower pressures and flow rates are sufficient for adequate visualization compared to abdominal laparoscopy. The remaining attachments to the uterus are on either lateral side. The laparoscope is introduced into the retractor, most frequently either a 0° or 30° 10 mm scope is used. A vessel sealing device is most commonly used along with a grasping instrument that may be a cautery instrument as well. Beginning on the patient's left side, the cervix is pushed medially and cephalad to give direct visualization of the uterine vessels. These are cauterized and cut followed by resection of the broad ligament up to the fundus. The round ligament can be transected, but the adnexal attachments remain in place until completion of dissection of the right side.

Attention is then focused on the right side of the uterus where the cervix is again manipulated medially and cranially and the uterine vessels are secured. One dissects the broad ligament of the right side and then one can resect both the round ligament and the adnexa (or utero-ovarian pedicle if the adnexa is to be preserved). Finally the left adnexa are managed in a similar fashion. This will free the uterus of all its attachments and it can be delivered through the vagina. Any portion of the tubes and ovaries can be removed with the uterus. The abdomen is then explored and ancillary procedures can be performed if necessary including omentectomy, peritoneal biopsies, appendectomy, lysis of adhesions, or umbilical hernia repair to name a few. As with abdominal laparoscopy any concern for specimen spill can be avoided with the use of endoscopic bags.

In some circumstances surgeons will perform a total vaginal NOTES whereby the retractor is placed into the vagina and circumcision of the cervix, entry into the anterior and posterior cul-de-sac, and the remainder the procedure are all performed by laparoscopic techniques through the vagina without placing the retractor into the peritoneal cavity. This technique may be helpful in women with a very high cervix (no descent) or a narrowed vagina such as may occur in post-menopausal or virginal women.

VNOTES techniques can also be utilized for adnexal surgery without removal of the uterus. In this situation an incision is made in the posterior cul-de-sac of the vagina between the uterosacral ligaments. A smaller Alexis retractor is then placed into the posterior cul-de-sac through which the laparoscope and instruments are introduced and surgery performed. This can be used for salpingectomy, oophorectomy, ovarian cystectomy, resection of ectopic pregnancy, or myomectomy.

5. Instrumentation for vNOTES

The instruments for performing vNOTES are similar to those used with transabdominal single incision laparoscopy. The V-Path Alexis retractor (Applied Medical, Rancho Santa Margarita, CA) has been approved by the FDA specifically for this procedure. Most surgeons utilize a 10 mm laparoscope. Because the field of surgery is so close to the retractor, the camera does not interfere with the other instruments and the larger aperture produces better lighting and visualization. A 0° or a 30° scope can be used depending on individual preference. Alternatively, some surgeons have access to 3D laparoscopes which provide better depth of field. Flexible laparoscopes do not appear to be advantageous for this procedure as they often collide with the pelvic tissues. Other instruments utilized during vNOTES include a vessel sealing instrument, a bipolar cautery instrument, and a grasping instrument such as a laparoscopic Maryland forcep depending on the individual surgeon's preference. Endoscopic bags can be used for specimen retrieval. Smoke evacuators and suction/irrigation are rarely necessary with the vNOTES approach as blood loss is generally minimal and smoke rarely interferes with visualization. The operative costs are no different than a standard single-incision laparoscopy.

6. Contraindications to vNOTES

Most contraindications to vNOTES must be considered relative based on the expertise of the surgeon. If one considers contraindications to abdominal laparoscopic surgery 20 years ago (prior surgery, endometriosis, obesity) one sees that with the evolution of techniques these are no longer applicable. Factors such as parity, prior cesarean delivery, lack of uterine descent, uterine size and concern for malignancy are not necessarily contraindications to vNOTES procedures. Most surgeons would avoid operating on women who have had low colorectal surgery, known obliteration of the posterior cul-de-sac, or prior pelvic radiation to reduce the risk of injury with the posterior entry. In addition, cervical myomas, depending on the position and size, may contribute to anatomic difficulties in placement of the retractor.

7. Current applications

7.1 Hysterectomy

Over 400 hysterectomies performed by vNOTES have been reported in the literature since 2012. There is a global registry that has currently amassed about 1800 cases from 40 vNOTES surgeons around the world with the majority including hysterectomy. Virtually any uterine pathology has undergone vNOTES hysterectomy including uteri greater than 2000 g. Uterine descent is not necessary for this procedure nor is prior cesarean delivery a contraindication. This approach can be used in morbidly obese women who will experience the most benefit from not having an abdominal incision. Myomectomy can also be performed from a vNOTES approach utilizing either the anterior or posterior cul-de-sac depending on the anatomic location of the myoma. Again the procedure itself is identical to that performed using transabdominal laparoscopy. The attached **video 1** demonstrates a vNOTES hysterectomy with bilateral salpingectomy.

7.2 Adnexal surgery

In women who wish to preserve their uterus but have an adnexal mass, vNOTES can be performed through the posterior cul-de-sac. The adnexal surgery may include removal of the fallopian tubes for sterilization, resection of ectopic pregnancy, ovarian cystectomy, or salpingo-oophorectomy. It is also possible to utilize this approach for diagnostic laparoscopy. This saves the patient from an abdominal incision and reduces the postoperative pain. The attached **video 2** demonstrates removal of an adnexal mass while leaving the uterus in place.

7.3 Pelvic support

Support of the vaginal cuff can be readily achieved through vNOTES. At the completion of the hysterectomy the visualization of the ureters permits very high plication of the uterosacral ligaments. An excellent demonstration of this technique can be seen in the following video by Dr. Howard Salvay https://www.youtube.com/watch?v=yYyPvuXEbxg. Sacrocolpopexy can also be performed using vNOTES, as demonstrated in a published series of 26 cases with correction of significant pelvic organ prolapse utilizing a Y-mesh to placate the sacral promontory to the anterior and posterior upper vagina [12]. This resulted in excellent postoperative results though long-term follow-up is still pending.

7.4 Additional gynecologic procedures

This approach is ideal for risk-reducing surgery in that the entire ovary and fallopian tube can be removed with a portion of the infundibulopelvic ligament and a pelvic washing for cytology can be obtained. In standard transvaginal surgery for adnexectomy adequate visualization to safely remove the entire tube and ovary is not always possible. The vNOTES approach also avoids an abdominal scar for a prophylactic surgery.

7.5 Non-gynecologic procedures

In most circumstances laparoscopic appendectomy is a relatively straight-forward procedure and can be safely accomplished by a vNOTES approach. Abdominal wall adhesions can be visualized and safely taken down which may alleviate some patients' symptoms of abdominal discomfort. Small umbilical hernias can be closed primarily or repaired with mesh against the abdominal wall through this approach.

8. Oncology applications

8.1 Endometrial cancer

Women with endometrial cancer are often obese and have multiple medical comorbidities. There are many reports of performing transvaginal hysterectomy on those patients who may not tolerate an abdominal procedure. However, that approach does not always permit visualization and removal of the tubes and ovaries. Nor does it allow for sampling of the lymph nodes. VNOTES permits removal of the tubes and ovaries, a pelvic washing can be performed, the entire abdomen can be explored, and lymph nodes can be removed. Multiple reports in the literature document the ability to perform Sentinel lymph nodes by this approach as well as pelvic lymphadenectomy and even aortic lymphadenectomy [13–16]. Given that the recommendation currently for staging endometrial cancer is to utilize a minimally invasive technique, vNOTES can provide an additional method to achieve this goal.

8.2 Ovarian cancer

In general ovarian cancer debulking is not performed with a minimally invasive technique; however, there are exceptions. When patients are treated with neo-adjuvant chemotherapy and have an excellent response, robotic or laparoscopic approach can be performed to remove any small residual disease. Early stage disease can also be staged by a minimally invasive route. A vNOTES approach can remove adnexal masses, the omentum, lymph nodes, and perform a full exploration of the abdominal cavity. The diaphragm can be reached with the appropriate instruments through the vagina to perform biopsies and visualization. Bulky disease in the pelvis would be a contraindication to a vNOTES approach as the likelihood of successfully entering the pouch of Douglas will be low.

8.3 Cervical cancer

There are no reports in the literature currently on utilizing vNOTES to treat cervical cancer. Theoretically a radical vaginal hysterectomy could be performed with vNOTES and pelvic lymph nodes can be removed so it is only a matter of time before some surgeons become skilled enough at this technique to perform such an operation. While there is currently controversy regarding a possible decreased survival with a minimally invasive radical hysterectomy [17], data on a radical vaginal approach does not appear to have a deleterious effect on outcome [18].

9. Conclusions

vNOTES has been shown to be a safe and feasible alternative approach to most gynecologic procedures. The technique is still in its infancy and is analogous to the early use of laparoscopy for advanced gynecologic surgery. There are distinct advantages with this approach including decreased pain, shorter recovery, and optimal cosmetics over standard laparoscopy. There is no doubt that vNOTES will be adopted by the surgical field. Instrumentation specific for vNOTES is beginning to be brought to the marketplace. Patient satisfaction with the technique will also drive more surgeons to these procedures. With vNOTES a gynecologist is able to offer the best aspects of laparoscopy with the ideal approach through the vagina.

Video materials

Video 1. vNOTES hysterectomy with bilateral salpingectomy. https://youtu.be/RvQcZfWEKDc
Video 2. vNOTES adnexal removal. https://youtu.be/fVxE3tErnwU

Author details

Alexander F. Burnett[1]* and Martha O. Rojo[2]

1 Division of Gynecologic Oncology, University of Arkansas for Medical Sciences, Little Rock, Arkansas, United States

2 UAMS School of Nursing, University of Arkansas for Medical Sciences, Little Rock, Arkansas, United States

*Address all correspondence to: aburnett@uams.edu

IntechOpen

References

[1] Decker A, Cherry TH. Culdopscopy: a new method in the diagnosis of pelvic disease – preliminary report. Am J Surgery 1944; 64:40-44

[2] Wright JD, Herzog TJ, Tsui J, Ananth CV, Lewin SN, Lu YS, et al. Nationwide trends in the performance of inpatient hysterectomy in the United States. Obstet Gynecol 2013;122:233-241.

[3] ACOG Committee Opinion 701. Choosing the route of hysterectomy for benign disease. *Committee Opinion 701.* June 2017

[4] AAGL position statement: route of hysterectomy to treat benign uterine disease. *JMIG* 2011; 18: 1-2

[5] Zorron R, Filgueiras M, Maggioni LC, Pombo L, Lopes Carvalho G, Lacerda Oliveira A. NOTES. Transvaginal cholecystectomy: report of the first case. Surg Innov 2007; 14P: 279-283

[6] Ahn KH, Song JY, Kim SH, Lee KW, Kim T. Transvaginal single-port natural orifice transluminal endoscopic surgery for benign uterine adnexal pathologies. JMIG 2012; 631-635

[7] Su H, Yen C, Wu K, Han C, Lee C. Hysterectomy via transvaginal natural orifice transluminal endoscopic surgery (NOTES): Feasibility of an innovative approach. Taiwaese J Ob Gyn 2012; 217-221

[8] Baekelandt J. Total vaginal NOTES hysterectomy: a new approach to hysterectomy. JMIG 2015a; 22: 1088-1094

[9] Baekelandt J. Total vaginal NOTES hysterectomy: a new approach to hysterectomy.JMIG 2015b; 22: 1088-1094

[10] Baekelandt JF, De Mulder PA, Le Roy I, Mathieu C, Laenen A, Enzlin P, Weyers S, Mol, BWJ, Bosteels JJA.

Hysterectomy by transvaginal natural orifice transluminalendoscopic surgery versus laparoscopy as a day-care procedure: a randomized controlled trial. BJOG 2019a; 26, 105-113

[11] Baekelandt JF, De Mulder PA, Le Roy I, Mathieu C, Laenen A, Enzlin P, Weyers S, Mol BWJ, Bosteels JJA. Hysterectomy by transvaginal natural orifice transluminal endoscopic surgery versus laparoscopy as a day-care procedure: a randomized controlled trial. BJOG 2019b; 126: 105-113

[12] Liu J, Kohn J, Fu H, Guan Z, Guan X. Transvaginal natural orifice transluminal endoscopic surgery for sacrocolpopexy: a pilot study of 26 cases. JMIG 2019; 748-753

[13] Baekelandt JF. New retroperitoneal transvaginal natural orifice transluminal endoscopic surgery approach to sentinel lymph node for endometrial cancer: demonstration video. JMIG 2019a; 26, 1231-1232

[14] Baekelandt JF. New retroperitoneal transvaginal natural orifice transluminal endoscopic surgery approach to sentinel node for endometrial cancer: a demonstration video. JMIG 2019b; 26: 1231-1232

[15] Leblanc E, Narducci F, Bresson L, Hudry D. Fluorescence-assisted sentinel (SND) and pelvic node dissections by single-p[ort transvaginal laparoscopic surgery, for the management of an endometrial carcinoma (EC)in an elderly obese patient. Gyn Onc 2016; 686-687

[16] Tantitamit T, Lee CL. Application of sentinel lymph node technique to transvaginal natural orifice transluminal endoscopic surgery in endometrial cancer. JMIG 2019; 626, 949-953

[17] Ramirez PT, Frumovitz M, Pareja R, Lopez A, Vieira M et al. Minimally

invasive versus abdominal radical hysterectomy for cervical cancer. NEJM 2018;379: 1905-1914

[18] Zhang S, Ma L, Meng QW, Zhou D, Moyiding T. Comparison of laparoscopic-assisted radical vaginal hysterectomy and abdominal radical hysterectomy in patients with early stage cervical cancer, a retrospective study. *Medicine* 2017; 96: 36

www.ingramcontent.com/pod-product-compliance
Lightning Source LLC
Chambersburg PA
CBHW081235190326
41458CB00016B/5792